Cleft Lip and/ or Palate Q & A

Nagato Natsume

Cleft Lip and/ or Palate Q & A

Edited by : NAGATO NATSUME

This book was originally published in Japanese under the title of :

KOUSHIN KOUGAIRETSU Q & A 140 (Cleft Lip and Palate : 140 Qs and As)

Natsume Nagato et al.

©2015 1st ed. ISHIYAKU PUBLISHERS, INC.

7-10, Honkomagome 1 chome, Bunkyo-ku,

Tokyo 113-8612, Japan

All rights reserved. This book or any part may not be reproduced, stored in a system, or transmitted in any form or any means, electric, mechanical, photocopying, recording, or otherwise without prior written permission from publisher.

Printed by NEOMEDIX CO., LTD

5-22-28 Chiyoda, Naka-ku Nagoya 460-0012, Japan

Tel: +81-052-241-7428

FAX: +81-052-241-7959

Edited and Sold by NAGASUESHOTEN., LTD

69-2 Itsutsujicho, Kamigyo-ku, Kyoto 602-8446, Japan

Tel: +81-075-415-7280

FAX: +81-075-415-7290

19 March 2025

ISBN 978-4-8160-1449-9 C3047 ￥2546

JSPS KAKENHI Grant Number 23HP6002

Preface

It has been more than 40 years since I decided to make cleft lip and palate treatment my lifework.

During those years, medical care regarding cleft lip and palate has made great strides, and I myself have learned a great deal through my clinical work. In the process, patients and their families have asked me many questions. Many of those questions were common, and I thought that if patients and their families could get the answers to those questions, it would alleviate some of their concerns. That is the reason why I have designed this book.

This book is intended to answer as many of these questions as possible, but they are not complete nor sufficient in many cases. Please be aware that some of the information in this document is my personal views.

Some of the contents of this book are based on our research supported by JSPS Grants-in-Aid for Scientific Research. Those studies were entitled "Genetic analysis research related to oral congenital anomalies" (2004-2006: 16209060), "Study concerning analysis of genes causing oral congenital anomalies" (2007-2010: 19209062), "Genomic analysis of genes relating to oral and maxillofacial congenital anomalies - Establishing a center of human genome resource banking" (2012-2018: 24249092) (Principal Investigator: Nagato Natsume), and the "Challenging attempts of prevention of certain cleft palate only: An idea for clinical application of epidemiological results" (2013-2015: 25670866, 2016-2018: 16K15830) (Principal Investigator: Nagato Natsume).

Finally, I would like to express my sincere gratitude to Mr. Fumio Kawaguchi, the former president of the Japanese Cleft Palate Foundation (JCPF), and Mr. Akihisa Mizuno, President of JCPF, Mr. Kenko Tatsuya, Chairman of Aichi Gakuin Educational Corporation, and Prof. Bunki Kimura, President of Aichi Gakuin University for their support in publishing this book. I also extend my gratitude to Dr. Ariuntuul Garidkhuu, Dr. Tselmuun Chinzorig, Ms. Oyunaa Erdene and Dr. Duurenjargal Myagmarsuren for translating this book. Lastly, I sincerely thank Mr. Hideki Nagasue for his total support as the publisher of this book.

Nagato Natsume
Professor, Cleft Lip and Palate Center, Aichi Gakuin University
Professor, Division of Research and Treatment for Oral and Maxillofacial Congenital
Anomalies, School of Dentistry, Aichi Gakuin University
Executive Director, Japanese Cleft Palate Foundation (JCPF)
Chairperson/Secretary/Treasurer, International Cleft Lip and Palate Foundation (ICPF)

CONTENTS

CHAPTER 1. BASIC INFORMATION ABOUT CLEFT LIP AND PALATE

Q 1. WHAT IS A CLEFT LIP? ·· 2

Q 2. DOES THE FETUS HAVE CLEFT LIP DURING DEVELOPMENT? ·············· 2

Q 3. WHAT SYNDROMES ARE ASSOCIATED WITH CLEFT LIP AND PALATE? ····· 3

Q 4. WHAT IS A SYNDROME? ·· 3

Q 5. WHAT IS THE CAUSE OF CLEFT LIP AND PALATE? ····························· 5

Q 6. CAN CLEFT LIP AND PALATE BE PREVENTED? ································· 5

Q 7. HOW ABOUT TAKING MEDICINES DURING PREGNANCY? ················ 6

Q 8. WHAT IS THE RELATIONSHIP BETWEEN THE ENVIRONMENT AND CLEFT LIP
AND PALATE? ·· 8

Q 9. PLEASE EXPLAIN ABOUT RELATIONSHIP BETWEEN THE MENTAL AND
PHYSICAL STATE OF EXPECTANT MOTHERS AND CLEFT LIP/PALATE ······· 9

Q 10. HOW TO GET GENETIC COUNSELLING APPOINTMENT (IN JAPAN)? ········ 11

Q 11. PLEASE TELL US REGARDING GENETIC COUNSELING ··············· 12

Q 12. PLEASE EXPLAIN REGARDING PLANNED PREGNANCY? ················· 13

Q 13. PLEASE TELL ME ABOUT PRENATAL TESTING? ····························· 14

Q 14. IS JAPANESE MEDICAL TREATMENT BEHIND OTHER COUNTRIES? ········ 16

CHAPTER 2. PRE-SURGERY AND SURGERY

Q 15. WHAT SHOULD BE PREPARED BEFORE SURGERY? ······················ 18

Q 16. EVEN AFTER SURGERY, WILL THE CLEFT LIP OR PALATE STILL BE
NOTICEABLE? ·· 19

Q 17. PLEASE EXPLAIN THE TREATMENT AND SURGICAL PROCEDURES FOR
CLEFT LIP AND PALATE FROM INFANCY TO ADULTHOOD ····················· 19

Q 18. CAN YOU EXPLAIN THE SURGICAL PROCEDURE FOR CLEFT LIP REPAIR?
·· 22

Q 19. PLEASE TELL ABOUT CLEFT PALATE SURGERY ························· 27

Q 20. WHY CAN'T SURGERY BE DONE IMMEDIATELY AFTER BIRTH? ············ 30

Q 21. I HAVE BEEN TOLD THAT MY CHILD HAS A HEART CONDITION. CAN MY
CHILD STILL HAVE SURGERY FOR CLEFT LIP AND PALATE? ················· 31

Q 22. HOW MANY SURGERIES ARE NEEDED FOR CLEFT LIP AND PALATE? ······ 31

Q 23. PLEASE TELL ME ABOUT PREOPERATIVE CORRECTION FOR THE FIRST
SURGERY ·· 32

Q 24. CAN GENERAL ANESTHESIA CAUSE ANY OTHER PROBLEMS? ··············· 34

Q 25. WHAT ARE THE EFFECTS OF X-RAYS TAKEN FOR THE TREATMENT OF CLEFT LIP AND PALATE ON THE BODY? ·········· 35

Q 26. CAN I BORROW X-RAYS AND TEST RESULTS FROM THE FACILITY I AM CURRENTLY VISITING WHEN GETTING A SECOND OPINION AT ANOTHER FACILITY? ·········· 36

Q 27. HOW TO HELP YOUR CHILD GAIN WEIGHT BEFORE PALATE SURGERY ··· 37

Q 28. MY CHILD SUCKS THEIR THUMB. HOW CAN WE ADDRESS THIS BEFORE SURGERY? ·········· 39

Q 29. WHY IS VACCINATION BEFORE CLEFT LIP AND PALATE SURGERY RESTRICTED, AND HOW SHOULD POST-SURGERY VACCINATIONS BE MANAGED? ·········· 40

Q 30. WHEN HOSPITALIZED, IS IT BETTER TO HAVE A PRIVATE ROOM OR A SHARED ROOM? ·········· 42

Q 31. FREQUENTLY ASKED QUESTIONS: ARM RESTRAINTS ·········· 43

Q 32. IT HAS BEEN A MONTH SINCE MY CLEFT LIP SURGERY, BUT THE REDNESS OF MY SCARS HAS NOT FADED, AND I STILL HAVE VISIBLE SCARS. WHAT SHOULD I DO? ·········· 44

Q 33. PLEASE TELL ME HOW TO FEED MY CHILD AFTER CLEFT LIP SURGERY ·········· 45

Q 34. WHAT EFFECT DOES A RETAINER NOSTRIL HAVE? ·········· 45

Q 35. WHY IS A PROTECTIVE PLATE USED AFTER CLEFT PALATE SURGERY? ··· 47

Q 36. WHAT PRECAUTIONS SHOULD PARENTS TAKE AFTER THE CHILD IS DISCHARGED? ·········· 48

Q 37. WHAT IS VESTIBULOPLASTY, AND WHY IS IT PERFORMED? ·········· 50

Q 38. WHEN IS REVISION SURGERY FOR CLEFT LIP OR PALATE NECESSARY? ·········· 51

Q 39. WHAT TREATMENTS ARE AVAILABLE FOR PRESCHOOL AND SCHOOL-AGE CHILDREN? ·········· 52

Q 40. WHAT KIND OF TREATMENTS ARE AVAILABLE FOR HIGH SCHOOL AND COLLEGE STUDENTS? ·········· 55

Q 41. IS IT POSSIBLE TO PERFORM BONE GRAFTING OR DISTRACTION OSTEOGENESIS SIMULTANEOUSLY WITH REVISION SURGERY? ·········· 56

Q 42. PROVIDE INFORMATION ON THE ADVANTAGES AND DISADVANTAGES OF PHARYNGEAL FLAP SURGERY, INCLUDING THE PROCEDURE, RECOVERY TIME, AND POTENTIAL RISKS ·········· 57

Q 43. ALVEOLAR BONE GRAFTING, ADVANTAGES AND LIMITATIONS AND THE TIMING OF THE PROCEDURE ·········· 58

Q 44. WHAT IS ALVEOLAR CLEFT BONE GRAFTING? ·········· 59

Q 45. IS IT POSSIBLE TO PUT IMPLANTS IN REPLACEMENT BONES? PLEASE EXPLAIN THE ACTUAL METHOD? ·········· 60

v

CONTENTS

Q 46. IS IT POSSIBLE TO HAVE BONE GRAFTING FOR ADULTS? ·················· 61

Q 47. PLEASE SHARE ABOUT REGENERATIVE TREATMENT AND ITS ADVANTAGES DURING ALVEOLAR BONE TRANSPLANTATION ·················· 62

Q 48. CAN YOU TELL ME ABOUT THE TIME AND SURGICAL METHOD OF CLOSING PALATAL FISTULA? ·················· 63

Q 49. WOULD IT BE AVAILABLE FOR ADULTS, WHO HAS CROSSBITE TO BE TREATED? ·················· 64

Q 50. WHAT IS CORRECTIVE SURGERY? WHAT TYPES OF SURGERIES ARE EXIST? ·················· 65

Q 51. TELL US ABOUT WHAT IS BONE LENGTHENING SURGERY, ITS INSTRUMENTS AND METHODS AND TIME? ·················· 66

Q 52. IS IT POSSIBLE TO MAKE SCARS FROM CLEFT LIP SURGERY LESS NOTICEABLE? ·················· 67

CHAPTER 3. ORTHODONTICS, PROSTHODONTICS

Q 53. IS PATIENTS WITH CLEFTS SUSPECTED TO HAVE CROSSBITE? ·················· 70

Q 54. WILL A CHILD WITH CLEFT LIP AND PALATE DEVELOP TEETH MISALIGNMENT, AND IS ORTHODONTIC TREATMENT INEVITABLE? ·················· 71

Q 55. I WAS TOLD NOT TO LET MY CHILD GET CAVITIES FOR THE SAKE OF FUTURE ORTHODONTIC TREATMENT. WHY IS THAT? ·················· 75

Q 56. PLEASE PROVIDE INFORMATION ABOUT THE COST OF ORTHODONTIC TREATMENT AND AVAILABLE PUBLIC SUBSIDIES ·················· 77

Q 57. WHEN IS THE OPTIMAL TIME TO BEGIN ORTHODONTIC TREATMENT FOR CHILDREN WITH CLEFT LIP AND PALATE, AND HOW LONG WILL IT TAKE? ·················· 79

Q 58. SHOULD TEETH WITH ABNORMAL MORPHOLOGY OR MALPOSITION THAT HAVE ERUPTED IN THE CLEFT AREA BE EXTRACTED EARLY? ·················· 81

Q 59. DOES ORTHODONTIC TREATMENT CREATE OR ENLARGE A HOLE IN THE PALATE? ·················· 82

Q 60. PLEASE TELL ME ABOUT IMPLANTS FOR CLEFT LIP AND PALATE ·················· 83

Q 61. HOW SHOULD I PROCEED IF I NEED TO CHANGE ORTHODONTIC CLINICS DUE TO A TRANSFER? WHAT WILL HAPPEN TO THE TREATMENT COSTS UP UNTIL THAT POINT AND THE FUTURE COSTS? ·················· 88

CHAPTER 4. SPEECH, LANGUAGE

Q 62. PLEASE TELL ME ABOUT DEVELOPMENTAL AND PSYCHOLOGICAL TESTS ·················· 92

Q 63. FOR CHILDREN WITH A CLEFT LIP, IS THERE A POSSIBILITY OF SPEECH OR

LANGUAGE DISORDERS? ·· 94

Q 64. IF THE SURGERY FOR CLEFT LIP IS DELAYED, WILL IT AFFECT SPEECH AND
LANGUAGE? ·· 95

Q 65. IF A CHILD WITH A CLEFT PALATE IS DELAYED IN RECEIVING SURGERY
DUE TO LOW WEIGHT, WILL IT AFFECT THEIR LANGUAGE OR ACADEMIC
DEVELOPMENT IN THE FUTURE? ·· 96

Q 66. DO CHILDREN NEED SPEECH THERAPY AFTER CLEFT PALATE SURGERY?
·· 97

Q 67. PLEASE ADVISE ON WHAT TO BE MINDFUL OF REGARDING LANGUAGE AT
HOME BEFORE THE SURGERY ·· 98

Q 68. YOU WERE ADVISED NOT TO CORRECT THE PRONUNCIATION, BUT WHY IS
THAT? ·· 98

Q 69. AFTER CLEFT PALATE SURGERY, IS THERE ANY TRAINING THAT CAN BE
DONE AT HOME? ·· 100

Q 70. MY CHILD HAS A HOLE AFTER CLEFT PALATE SURGERY. WILL THIS AFFECT
THEIR SPEECH IN THE FUTURE? ·· 101

Q 71. PLEASE LET ME KNOW ABOUT SPEECH AND LANGUAGE TRAINING ······ 102

Q 72. WHAT IS VELOPHARYNGEAL DYSFUNCTION? ·· 106

Q 73. PLEASE TELL ME ABOUT HYPERNASALITY ·· 107

Q 74. WHAT IS ABNORMAL ARTICULATION? ·· 108

Q 75. WHAT CAN BE UNDERSTOOD FROM A FIBER SCOPE EXAMINATION? ······ 109

Q 76. WHAT CAN BE DETERMINED FROM A CEPHALOMETRIC EXAMINATION?
·· 111

Q 77. WHAT ARE SPEECH AIDS AND PALATAL LIFT PROSTHESES (PLP)? AND
WHEN ARE THEY USED? ·· 111

Q 78. DOES SURGERY ON THE ADENOIDS AFFECT SPEECH? ·· 113

Q 79. IS IT POSSIBLE FOR PRONUNCIATION TO WORSEN AFTER ENTERING
ELEMENTARY SCHOOL? ·· 114

Q 80. IF THERE IS AN ABNORMALITY IN PRONUNCIATION, COULD IT BE DUE TO
A CLEFT PALATE, EVEN IF THERE IS NO VISIBLE EXTERNAL ABNORMALITY?
·· 115

Q 81. I AM STRUGGLING WITH HOW TO COMMUNICATE WITH MY SON, WHO WAS
BORN WITH A CLEFT PALATE. AT ONE AND A HALF YEARS OLD, HE IS NOT
SAYING ANY WORDS OTHER THAN "MAMA" AND IS COMMUNICATING
THROUGH GESTURES AND SIGNS. WHAT SHOULD I DO? ································ 116

CHAPTER 5. CHILDCARE

Q 82. IS IT TRUE THAT CHILDREN WITH CLEFT LIP AND PALATE EXPERIENCE
SLOWER PHYSICAL GROWTH? ·· 118

vii

CONTENTS

Q 83. DOES A CHILD WITH CLEFT LIP AND PALATE EXPERIENCE DELAYED
SPEECH DEVELOPMENT, LEADING TO LOWER INTELLIGENCE OR SLOWER
MENTAL DEVELOPMENT? ·· 119

Q 84. ARE THERE ANY RESTRICTIONS FOR CHILDREN WITH CLEFT LIP AND
PALATE WHEN IT COMES TO SPORTS (E.G., ACTIVITIES THEY SHOULD
AVOID)? ALSO, ARE THERE ANY AREAS THEY MIGHT STRUGGLE WITH? ··· 120

Q 85. IS IT NECESSARY TO WRITE "CLEFT LIP AND PALATE" IN THE DISEASE
COLUMN OF THE PRE-VACCINATION MEDICAL QUESTIONNAIRE? ARE THERE
ANY PRECAUTIONS TO TAKE WHEN RECEIVING VACCINATIONS? ············· 121

Q 86. SHOULD I CONSULT WITH KINDERGARTEN OR SCHOOL TEACHERS? ····· 122

Q 87. HOW SHOULD I EXPLAIN THE POSTOPERATIVE SCAR TO MY CHILD? ····· 123

Q 88. HOW SHOULD I EXPLAIN TO MY CHILD'S FRIENDS? ···························· 124

Q 89. "I WOULD LIKE TO HEAR ABOUT THE EXPERIENCE OF RAISING A CHILD
WITH THE SAME CONDITION..." ··· 125

Q 90. "I WOULD LIKE TO CORRESPOND WITH MOTHERS OF CHILDREN WITH
CLEFT LIP AND PALATE ABROAD..." ·· 125

Q 91. ARE THERE ANY CLEFT LIP AN PALATE NGO'S OVERSEAS? ··················· 126

Q 92. DO CHILDREN WITH CLEFT LIP AND PALATE PASS GAS A LOT? ············· 126

Q 93. IS THERE A MOVIE TO HELP UNDERSTAND CLEFT LIP AND PALATE? ······ 127

CHAPTER 6. TREATMENT COST, SOCIAL SERVICES

Q 94. PLEASE TELL ME ABOUT THE INSURANCE SYSTEMS AVAILABLE FOR
PATIENTS WITH CLEFT LIP AND PALATE ··· 130

Q 95. WHAT PROCEDURES SHOULD BE APPLIED FOR AFTER THE BIRTH OF A
CHILD WITH A CLEFT LIP AND PALATE? ··· 130

Q 96. CAN YOU TELL ME ABOUT MEDICAL AID FOR SELF-RELIANCE?   DOES IT
MAKE MEDICAL EXPENSES FREE IF APPLIED?
ALSO, UNTIL WHAT AGE IS IT APPLICABLE? ·· 131

Q 97. WHAT IS THE COST OF THE FIRST AND CORRECTIVE SURGERIES?
ALSO, ARE THE MEDICAL AID FOR SELF-RELIANCE OR HEALTH INSURANCE
SYSTEMS APPLICABLE? ··· 131

Q 98. FOR INDIVIDUALS AGED 18 AND OLDER, WHAT IS THE COST OF
SECONDARY SURGERIES? ·· 132

Q 99. WHAT IS THE COST OF ORTHODONTIC TREATMENT, PROSTHETIC DENTAL
TREATMENT, AND IMPLANT TREATMENT? ALSO, ARE MEDICAL AID FOR
SELF-RELIANCE AND HEALTH INSURANCE SYSTEMS APPLICABLE? ········· 133

Q 100. WHAT IS THE COST OF SPEECH THERAPY? ALSO, ARE MEDICAL AID FOR
SELF-RELIANCE AND HEALTH INSURANCE SYSTEMS APPLICABLE? ········· 135

Q 101. CAN A DISABILITY CERTIFICATE BE RECEIVED IN THE CASE OF CLEFT LIP

AND PALATE? 136

Q 102. DOES OBTAINING A DISABILITY CERTIFICATE DISADVANTAGE YOU WHEN SEEKING EMPLOYMENT? 136

Q 103. WHAT IS A REHABILITATION HANDICAPPED PERSON'S HANDBOOK? ... 137

Q 104. WHY DO MEDICAL COST SUBSIDIES DIFFER BETWEEN MUNICIPALITIES? 137

Q 105. PLEASE TELL ME ABOUT THE EDUCATIONAL INSURANCE THAT CHILDREN WITH CLEFT LIP AND PALATE CAN GET 138

Q 106. PLEASE TELL ME ABOUT LIFE INSURANCE THAT CHILDREN WITH CLEFT LIP AND PALATE CAN ENROLL IN 138

Q 107. EVEN WITH A CONGENITAL DISEASE, IS IT POSSIBLE TO JOIN MEDICAL INSURANCE IN THE FUTURE? 139

CHAPTER 7. FEEDING PROBLEMS

Q 108. PLEASE TELL ME ABOUT FEEDING CHILDREN WITH CLEFT LIP AND PALATE 142

Q 109. WHEN SHOULD WE START INTRODUCING SOLID FOODS, AND HOW SHOULD WE PROCEED? 146

Q 110. PLEASE TELL ME ABOUT THE DIET (EATING HABITS) AFTER SURGERY FOR CLEFT LIP AND CLEFT PALATE. ALSO, WILL THE BABY BE ABLE TO BREASTFEED IMMEDIATELY AFTER THE SURGERY? 148

Q 111. CAN A 9-MONTH-OLD CHILD WITH A CLEFT PALATE DRINK FROM A STRAW? 149

Q 112. EVEN AFTER UNDERGOING CLEFT PALATE SURGERY, FOOD IS LEAKING FROM MY CHILD'S NOSE... 150

Q 113. WHAT IS ESOPHAGEAL REFLUX DISEASE? 151

CHAPTER 8. EAR PROBLEMS

Q 114. WHEN SHOULD WE START VISITING AN ENT (EAR, NOSE, AND THROAT) SPECIALIST? 154

Q 115. IS THERE ANYTHING TO BE AWARE OF FROM AN ENT PERSPECTIVE BEFORE THE SURGERY? 155

Q 116. PLEASE TELL ME ABOUT OTITIS MEDIA WITH EFFUSION 156

Q 117. I WOULD LIKE TO HAVE A HEARING TEST. FROM WHAT AGE IS IT POSSIBLE TO UNDERGO THE TEST? 160

Q 118. DOES HAVING A CLEFT PALATE AFFECT THE SENSE OF SMELL? 161

Q 119. IS IT TRUE THAT CHILDREN WITH CLEFT LIP AND PALATE HAVE A FOUL-SMELLING NOSE? 162

CONTENTS

CHAPTER 9. DENTAL PROBLEMS

Q 120. ARE CHILDREN WITH CLEFT LIP AND PALATE MORE PRONE TO CAVITIES? 164

Q 121. ARE THERE ANY SPECIAL CONSIDERATIONS WHEN BRUSHING THE TEETH OF CHILDREN WITH CLEFT LIP AND PALATE? COULD YOU ALSO EXPLAIN THE EFFECTIVENESS OF FLUORIDE IN PREVENTING CAVITIES? 165

Q 122. IS SEVERE TEETH GRINDING AFFECTING MY TEETH? IS THERE A WAY TO STOP IT? 168

Q 123. DOES GETTING CAVITIES AFFECT PRONUNCIATION? 169

Q 124. IS IT POSSIBLE TO APPLY FLUORIDE TREATMENT IN THE CASE OF CLEFT LIP AND PALATE? 170

Q 125. WILL A TOOTH GROW IN THE AREA WHERE THERE WAS A CLEFT? 171

Q 126. PLEASE TEACH ME HOW TO BRUSH TEETH IN THE AREA OF THE ALVEOLAR CLEFT 172

Q 127. IS IT EASIER TO DEVELOP PERIODONTAL DISEASE IF YOU HAVE A CLEFT LIP AND PALATE? 173

CHAPTER 10. PSYCHOLOGICAL PROBLEMS

Q 128. WHAT IS THE CONSULTATION AND TELEPHONE SUPPORT SYSTEM? 176

Q 129. WHEN SHOULD I CONSULT A CLINICAL PSYCHOLOGIST? 176

Q 130. HOW CAN BULLYING BE PREVENTED OR ERADICATED? 177

CHAPTER 11. OTHERS

Q 131. HOW DO THE GENERAL PUBLIC RECOGNIZE SPEECH DISORDERS RELATED TO CLEFT LIP AND CLEFT PALATE? 180

Q 132. IS IT POSSIBLE TO EXPERIENCE DISCRIMINATION DURING EMPLOYMENT OR MARRIAGE? 181

Q 133. WHEN A POTENTIAL PARTNER FOR MARRIAGE APPEARS, SHOULD YOU TELL THEM ABOUT YOUR CLEFT LIP AND PALATE? 181

Q 134. AS A PATIENT WITH CLEFT LIP AND PALATE, YOU MAY WANT TO HAVE A PARTNER OR GET MARRIED, BUT YOU MIGHT WORRY THAT YOUR APPEARANCE OR GENETIC CONCERNS WILL EVENTUALLY DISAPPOINT YOUR PARTNER, MAKING YOU FEEL THAT YOU CANNOT BE "THE BEST PARTNER" FOR THEM. WHAT SHOULD YOU DO? 182

Q 135. IF THE PERSON YOU DECIDED TO MARRY, OR THEIR FAMILY, HAS CLEFT LIP AND PALATE, AND YOU ARE CONSIDERING BREAKING OFF THE MARRIAGE DUE TO PARENTAL OPPOSITION, WHAT SHOULD YOU DO? 182

Q 136. I SAW A TV BROADCAST SHOWING CHILDREN FROM DEVELOPING

COUNTRIES WITH CLEFT LIPS, AND MY CHILD STARTED CRYING. IS IT
ETHICALLY ACCEPTABLE FOR TV STATIONS TO AIR SUCH FOOTAGE? ······· 183

Q 137. IT IS SOMETIMES SEEN THAT OLDER INDIVIDUALS HAVE SCARS ON THEIR
UPPER LIPS. IS IT POSSIBLE TO TREAT THIS EVEN NOW? ························ 183

Q 138. MY BOYFRIEND, WHO HAS A CLEFT LIP AND PALATE, INTERRUPTED HIS
TREATMENT WHEN HE WAS YOUNG, AND IS NOW 20 YEARS OLD. IT IS LIKELY
THAT SURGERY COULD IMPROVE HIS CONDITION, BUT HE IS NOT
UNDERGOING THE PROCEDURE. ADDITIONALLY, HE HAS POOR DENTAL
ALIGNMENT, CAVITIES, AND HAS RECENTLY STARTED TO NOTICE BAD
BREATH. WHAT SHOULD BE DONE? ··· 184

Q 139. PLEASE TELL ME ABOUT THE JAPANESE CLEFT PALATE FOUNDATION
··· 184

Q 140. PLEASE TELL ME ABOUT THE INTERNATIONAL CLEFT LIP AND PALATE
FOUNDATION: ICPF ·· 186

CHAPTER *1.*
BASIC INFORMATION ABOUT CLEFT LIP AND PALATE

CHAPTER 1. BASIC INFORMATION ABOUT CLEFT LIP AND PALATE

Q 1. WHAT IS A CLEFT LIP?

A **Cleft lip is a congenital malformation where the skin and muscles of the lips do not properly fuse at birth during the fetal development. In other words, it can happen when the tissues of the lip fail to completely unite.**

Cleft lip and palate are a congenital anomaly resulting from the incomplete fusion of facial tissues (for example: bone and muscles) during embryonic development, leading to variations in facial structure at birth. During that process, a cleft lip is developed when the tissues of the lip area fail to unite properly, resulting in an incorrect shape.

During embryonic development up to a specific fetal stage, the lips can be split, potentially resulting in different types of cleft lips.

Q 2. DOES THE FETUS HAVE CLEFT LIP DURING DEVELOPMENT?

A **A fetus's lips fully form between 6th to 8th weeks of pregnancy, but if the lips failed merging at that time, cleft lips can occur.**

In modern times, fetal abnormalities can be diagnosed through prenatal diagnostics. A baby originates from a single cell within the mother's womb and develops through numerous cell divisions. During early pregnancy, the organs including the face, hands, and feet are not fully developed.

The lips are fully formed from the 6th to the 8th weeks of pregnancy, but if the lips do not meet at that time, cleft lip may happen. Cleft palate occurs later than this. At about 10 weeks of pregnancy, the palate is formed from the both sides. The development of the palate divides the process of respiration into nasal breathing and oral breathing. If the palate is not fully fused from both the left and right sides, a cleft palate will develop.

Both cleft lip and cleft palate together occur at the beginning of pregnancy, when the size of the fetus is very small, often a few centimeters, during which most mothers do not even aware of their pregnancy. It's a time when you can't sense it.

2

Q 3. WHAT SYNDROMES ARE ASSOCIATED WITH CLEFT LIP AND PALATE?

A **There are several syndromes. Among them, a number of syndromes can be identified by diagnostic tests for genetic congenital abnormalities.**

Cleft lip and palate can result from a combination of several disorders. There are currently 154 types of syndromes including Pierre Robin syndrome, Down syndrome, Van der Woude syndrome, Treacher Collins syndrome, Orofaciodigital syndrome or oral-facial-digital syndrome, Ectrodactyly-ectodermal dysplasia-cleft syndrome or EEC syndrome, 1st and 2nd branchial arch syndromes, Cornelia de Lange syndrome, Kabuki syndrome, oropalatodactyly syndrome, 22q11 Velo-cardio-facial syndrome etc.

Q 4. WHAT IS A SYNDROME?

A **A syndrome is a group of several illnesses and disorders occurring simultaneously.**

There are cases where children with cleft lip and palate are born with birth defects in areas other than cleft lip and palate. This is referred to as a syndrome. There is no single cause and cleft lip and palate can be hereditary. If your child is born with other disorders besides cleft lip and palate, it is advisable to consult a specialist.

There are 60-100 variations of cleft lip and palate syndromes, and some of them are undiagnosed until the child grows up. Let's explain the most common of the above-mentioned syndromes.

Van der Woude syndrome

This syndrome includes cleft lip and palate, affects around 1 in 500-700 individuals in Japan, causing a serious issue. Among children with cleft lip and palate, approximately 0.5-2% also have Van der Woude syndrome. The syndrome is seen in roughly 1 in 75,000-100,000 individuals in the general population. It commonly appears as a congenital lower lip fistula, usually with two symmetrical fistulas or occasionally in the midline or on one side. The fistula's aperture is irregular and may consist of a displaying protuberance and no salivary glands are present. In some cases, there are condition where they secrete saliva.

Van der Woude syndrome is an autosomal dominant genetic condition resulting from a mutation

3

in the IRF6 gene. Although it is often inherited in a single gene pattern, it frequently appears unexpectedly within families. The syndrome presents in many forms, with cleft lip and palate and congenital lower lip fistula as the primary symptoms. Secondary symptoms may involve the submucosal cleft palate, syndactyly, hypodontia. Precise genetic diagnosis and counseling are essential, as minor symptoms can easily be overlooked.

Fistulectomy is commonly done during palatoplasty or lip repair surgery for congenital lower lip fistula, followed by treatment identical to that for general cleft lip and palate cases.

Basal Cell Nevus Syndrome

Basal cell nevus syndrome presents with several disorders, including cleft lip and palate and basal cell tumors. Due to its diverse manifestations, it can be difficult to diagnose accurately. Genetic counseling, genetic testing, and imaging tests are advised for diagnosis. Despite being difficult to diagnose in the past without specialist intervention, genetic testing holds potential for more reliable future diagnoses. Timely detection via routine examinations and health check-ups can lead to in immediate treatment.

Seeking guidance from an expert is crucial for precise diagnosis, particularly for persons with cleft lip/palate and above syndrome disorders.

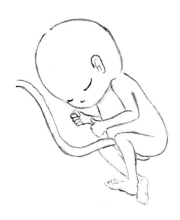

Q 5. WHAT IS THE CAUSE OF CLEFT LIP AND PALATE?

A Various factors contribute to the causes of cleft lip and palate.

It is commonly believed that cleft lip and palate are caused solely by genetic factors, but this is a major misconception. The exact cause is still unknown. It is important to note that while genetics play a role, various environmental factors are also involved.

For instance, in our animal research laboratory, we have subjected pregnant animals to conditions including food deprivation, sedatives, exposed to bacterial infections and other environmental factors. Results showed that those elements may result offspring with cleft lip and palate. Moreover, a deficiency in folic acid has been linked to this anomaly.

Thus, the most accepted theory on etiology of cleft lip and palate among researchers is multifactorial origin. Rather than a single cause of the disorder, it occurs when various factors are combined, including environmental and genetic. Some study mention that even obesity and diabetes might be one of the reasons, so in this sense cleft lip and palate is not a special disease. Although mutation of candidate genes has been discovered, the genetic relationship remains unknown for cause of cleft lip and palate.

Q 6. CAN CLEFT LIP AND PALATE BE PREVENTED?

A As of now, there is no known particular method to prevent cleft lip and palate, because the exact cause remains unknown.

There is no recognized method to prevent cleft lip and palate, as the exact cause remains unknown. Although some environmental factors are known, it is practically impossible to protect against all potential causes in our everyday life. Stress and hormonal changes in the body may also contribute to the development of this malformations.

Those who are planning to have a baby, before pregnancy consider genetic blood testing before conception, prioritize a healthy lifestyle, adequate nutrition and minimize stress as much as possible.

To date, we are actively engaged in research to discover evidence-based preventative techniques for cleft lip and palate within grants provided by the Ministry of Education, Culture, Sports, Science and Technology of Japan. We have published some results of the studies separately.

CHAPTER 1. BASIC INFORMATION ABOUT CLEFT LIP AND PALATE

Q 7. HOW ABOUT TAKING MEDICINES DURING PREGNANCY?

A Let's discuss about some groups of medications.

Cold medicines

A variety of chemicals are found in over-the-counter medications.

It often contains lysozyme chloride as an expectorant and anti-inflammatory enzyme component, dihydrocodeine phosphate as a cough suppressant and tracheal dilator, and acetaminophen as an antipyretic.

It is known that children and infants do not have any negative effects when taken orally, and the amount contained in cold medicine is not very high.

Psychiatric medications

Maternal mental status is known to affect the fetus. Mental instability can negatively impact the mother's lifestyle and nutritional habits, leading to a worsening of the prenatal environment and potentially influencing the fetus. It is important to contact with an obstetrician and gynecologist before stopping oral medication for mental illnesses.

The potential teratogenic consequences of oral medications for mental illnesses make them restricted and need to be used with caution. Talking to your doctor about getting pregnant before getting pregnant is crucial if you are currently undergoing treatment at a psychosomatic or psychiatric facility.

Steroids

Steroids are effective treatments for numerous illnesses. It is used in steroid ointments for atopic dermatitis, as well as for treating asthma, thyroid disease, and rheumatism.

However, there have been numerous reports of teratogenic effects caused by high dosages of steroids in animal studies. It is advisable to consult your doctor or obstetrician before discontinuing or decreasing the dosage to avoid potential complications with the pregnancy.

Oral medications are essential for the treatment of the disease, and it is crucial to refrain from making arbitrary adjustments, discontinuing medications, or adjusting dosages independently. Particularly, the fetus is not significantly affected by the medication, even if it is taken prior to pregnancy, provided that it is administered orally and does not produce any residual effects. This also applies to males.

Typically, if you become pregnant while taking medication, the critical period that could impact the fetus is the second month of pregnancy (fourth week of pregnancy). It is important to be aware of the phase of absolute hypersensitivity (weeks 4-7 of pregnancy) and the period of relative hypersensitivity following that (weeks 8-16 of pregnancy), as they are believed to have a greater impact on the fetus. Avoid taking the pill after ovulation in the menstrual cycle you want to conceive if you wish to be very cautious, always seek advice from your obstetrician before using any medicine while pregnant.

It is crucial to never cease, alter, or modify any medication alone and to always get advice from your obstetrician. If the pharmacological effect of the medication is thought to be greater than the side effects, you may be recommended to continue taking it, but stopping the medication of your own may worsen your symptoms and affect your fetus.

Not all nutrients, over-the-counter supplements are safe for pregnant women, and some may be harmful to the unborn baby if consumed excessively, such as vitamin A.

Make sure to discuss your obstetrician-gynecologist regarding the efficacy and potential adverse effects of any medicine.

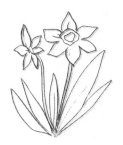

CHAPTER 1. BASIC INFORMATION ABOUT CLEFT LIP AND PALATE

Q 8. WHAT IS THE RELATIONSHIP BETWEEN THE ENVIRONMENT AND CLEFT LIP AND PALATE?

A **There is no definitive link between the concentration of soluble bisphenol A in daily life and cleft lip and palate. It is thought that the pollution levels in the average Japanese environment are not sufficiently high to cause cleft lip and palate.**

Things that directly or indirectly affect humans or other living things are referred to as environmental influences. These are commonly referred to as "hormones" of the environment. Two common examples of things we encounter on a daily basis are dioxin, which is found in the environment, and bisphenol A, which is used as a raw material for plastics. Let's discuss the connection between these chemicals and cleft lip and palate in this chapter.

Bisphenol A

Bisphenol A (BPA) is a chemical compound utilized in the production of polycarbonate containers such as plastic cups, pasta dishes, and infant bottles, as well as in the coating of canned goods. In 1988, concerns about BPA arose, prompting a risk assessment by the European Commission in 2003, which concluded that there were no negative impacts on the environment or human health. However, BPA was prohibited in infant bottles in 2011.

Japan has established a safety threshold for BPA in plastic bottles at 2.5 ppm according to the Food Sanitation Act. The level of BPA leaching out is even less than the amount contained in plastic food containers is lower than that expected, indicating no immediate health hazards. Research suggests that usual exposure levels of BPA in pregnant women and infants are not dangerous, despite concerns about its effects. There is no apparent link between BPA and cleft lip and palate, so there is no need to worry.

Dioxin

Dioxins are not naturally produced but are created by the combustion of different elements. When trash is burned, it releases dioxins into the air, which can build up in the soil, water, and creatures. Dioxins are commonly present in lipids, fish, meat, dairy products, and eggs because of their fat-soluble characteristics.

In Japan, the Department of Environmental Affairs conducted a survey in the 2011 fiscal year and determined that the groundwater quality and atmospheric dioxin levels met environmental criteria, measuring at 0.028 pg/m^3. Pollution levels have greatly reduced in the last ten years.

Animal studies have demonstrated cleft palates in pregnant mice exposed to dioxins, but it is thought that the current pollution levels in the normal environment in Japan do not have high amounts of dioxin pollution to cause cleft lip and palate. Due to differing eating patterns among individuals,

8

the most effective way to avoid cleft lip and palate is by adhering to a nutritious and balanced diet.

[Q] 9. PLEASE EXPLAIN ABOUT RELATIONSHIP BETWEEN THE MENTAL AND PHYSICAL STATE OF EXPECTANT MOTHERS AND CLEFT LIP/PALATE

[A] **Cleft lip/and or palate are not caused by a single factor but rather the result of a mix of multiple variables, making it a multifactorial disorder. Pregnant women must prioritize monitoring diseases like anemia and aim to maintain a stress-free lifestyle.**

If a pregnant woman has a worry

Stress can affect the body in several manners, particularly during gestation. Stress induces stimulation of the hypothalamus, resulting in a cascade of hormone releases and physiological reactions, including diminished lymphocytes and thyroid gland atrophy.

Stress can impact the development of the fetal nervous system and increase the likelihood of low birth weight and asthma. Cleft lip and palate are not attributable to a singular cause; rather, they are multifactorial conditions resulting from the interplay of various elements, indicating that stress alone does not induce them. Nonetheless, stress can be challenging for pregnant women; therefore, seek methods to manage your situation.

Strategies include sharing concerns with family, friends, and healthcare professionals, and participating in activities such as yoga, aerobics or swimming, can aid in lowering stress levels.

If pregnant mother has a hay fever

Effective management of hay fever symptoms is crucial for pregnant women. Hay fever does not directly impact the fetus, but persistent nasal congestion and itchy eyes might cause general weakness and depression. It is recommended to seek advice from an obstetrician about safe drugs, such as anti-allergy pills and eye drops.

If pregnant mother has anemia

Anemia in a pregnant woman indicates a reduction in the proportion of red blood cells in her blood. Throughout pregnancy, the need for blood rises as the fetus develops, resulting in a natural increase in the mother's total blood volume. If the rate of volume rise exceeds the formation of red blood cells, it leads to diluted blood, causing anemia. Approximately 30% of pregnant women will get anemia at some stage of their pregnancy. Blood is essential for transporting oxygen and nutrients to both the mother and the developing fetus. An anemic mother may affect the vital flow of oxygen and nutrients to the baby, which could result in delayed fetal growth and a higher likelihood of delivery problems.

If anemia continues beyond the second trimester and dietary changes are not effective, iron supplements may be advised. Pregnant women should prioritize a healthful diet as soon as they confirm their pregnancy.

Untreated anemia during pregnancy may lead to a higher occurrence of cleft lip and palate patients, according to data.

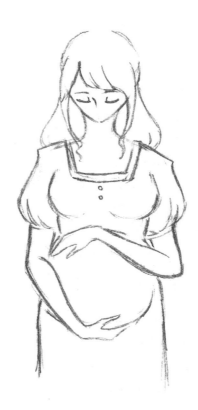

Q 10. HOW TO GET GENETIC COUNSELLING APPOINTMENT (IN JAPAN)?

A **For genetic counseling on cleft lip and palate, first you have to give a call to the center before booking a visit.**

First:

① Please contact (052) 757-4312 to make an appointment.

*Specify "genetic counseling" while making a call. A professional will contact you using the number you provided.

② Thorough Explanation during consultation

If you need clarification or genetic counseling, please refer your doctor.

Second:

③ Initial Encounter: Interview Summary

・Familial medical history (e.g. occurrence of similar congenital disorders in family members)・ Patient Medical History

Discussion about personal, familial, and related questions;

Subjects covered are genetic counseling, fertility consultation, pregnancy advise, explanation about congenital anomalies, genetic testing, and more.

- About "Prevention Programs" and other related topics to be known by patient;

Upon request, blood tests and consultations can be scheduled at Nagoya University Taiko Medical Center and Aichi Gakuin University Cleft Center based on the test results. Additional fees may be incurred.

④ Submitting a Counseling Application *Note: Expect a long wait period due to high demand.

⑤ Counseling Session *Scheduling in advance is essential. Currently, the estimated waiting period is 2-3 months.

Duration of consultation: 1 hour per person;

Consultation Fee: 2,500 JPY for a 20-minute session (self-pay). Separate consultations will be provided for married couples. (Counseling usually takes place on a one-on-one basis.) *Both parties might choose to have consultations on different days or at different times, if they request.

⑥ Second Visit

During the second visit a clinical geneticist will give you consultation. You can request a third visit.

⑦ Consultation completed.

CHAPTER 1. BASIC INFORMATION ABOUT CLEFT LIP AND PALATE

Q 11. PLEASE TELL US REGARDING GENETIC COUNSELING

A **Patients receive comprehensive analyses and precise explanations of their genetic information and family history during genetic counseling.**

It is well acknowledged that genes have a major role in determining characteristics like height, temperament, and the color of the skin and hair. Chromosome and genetic alterations, as well as roughly ten genetic alterations in autosomal recessive disorders, are considered to be inherited even in healthy people. It is estimated that 5-6% of newborns have morphological and functional anomalies that are discovered right away after delivery, including modest cases of endocrine disorders, serious heart disease, and cleft lip and palate. Numerous articles discuss these illnesses, their causes, and the results of genetic testing. The practice of giving people different information and explaining it to them is known as genetic counseling. Doctors explain professional information and complicated technical terms in a way that is suited for individuals and families, as many people find it difficult to understand them.

Clinical geneticists frequently provide genetic counseling, however big hospital genetics departments and general care physicians may also be consulted.

Q 12. PLEASE EXPLAIN REGARDING PLANNED PREGNANCY?

A The definition of "planned pregnancy" in medical contexts is "the process of preparing the mother's body and surroundings for the best possible outcomes for the fetus and the mother."

Although the term "planned pregnancy" is commonly used to refer to the scheduling and management of the delivery period, in medical terms it refers to situations where the mother's health necessitates extensive pre-pregnancy planning.

For example, it is crucial for pregnant women with diabetes to take care of their own health because severe reductions in blood sugar levels and deterioration of kidney function may occur after pregnancy. For instance, an insulin injection may be able to improve the condition even if it is adequately managed with oral medicine.

Carefully monitoring blood sugar levels is essential, as is making sure the family knows what to do if blood sugar levels fall. Therefore, it's crucial to plan your pregnancy not just to determine when to give birth, but also to ensure that you have enough medical care for any illnesses and that your family is aware of the situation beforehand.

Similarly, it is also considered planned pregnancy if you assess your lifestyle before to becoming pregnant, treat any chronic illnesses, and improve symptoms like anemia.

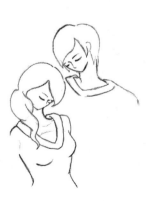

CHAPTER 1. BASIC INFORMATION ABOUT CLEFT LIP AND PALATE

Q 13. PLEASE TELL ME ABOUT PRENATAL TESTING?

A **A variety of techniques that enable the evaluation of fetal health are included in prenatal diagnostics. If necessary, please consult your doctor.**

The probability of miscarriage during amniocentesis and the types of diseases that can be detected by amniocentesis

The fluid that leaks out of the amniotic sac in the early phases of pregnancy is known as amniotic fluid. It is composed of plasma from the mother's and the infant's blood. Half of the amniotic fluid is replaced daily in the later stages of pregnancy by the baby's urination and consumption of amniotic fluid. In addition to acting as a cushion and shielding the unborn child from shocks, amniotic fluid provides nutrients essential for the healthy growth and development of the child.

An ultrasound is used during amniocentesis to guide the placement of a needle to remove 10-15 milliliters of amniotic fluid and to confirm the baby's and placenta's positions. Although miscarriages and stillbirths are the most common causes of the most significant side effects, it is estimated that only one out of every 300 to 500 women who have amniocentesis is a direct result of the procedure. A typical adverse effect is "rupture of the amniotic puncture," which is the release of amniotic fluid from the puncture site. But in the majority of situations, medication and hospitalization under a doctor's diagnosis will lead to recovery.

The collected amniotic fluid can be used to determine the baby's actual status. This enables to do chromosomal and genetic tests on the infant and to determine whether infectious illnesses are present. Some disorders may be challenging to identify and don't always produce conclusive, 100% results, like Down syndrome. Genetic testing is also available, targeting specific illnesses like hemophilia; nevertheless, it should be carefully evaluated and discussed with a healthcare physician. Before undergoing prenatal diagnostic testing, genetic counseling is the best way to completely understand the implications and make an informed decision.

The ultrasound appearance of cleft lip and palate

Cleft lip presence or absence can be properly recognized by ultrasound imaging. However, the fetal positioning—which is frequently typified by a rounded back—may obstruct the view of the limbs, making them invisible on the ultrasound scan.

The movement of the tongue inside the cleft during the ingestion of amniotic fluid may give the impression that a baby with a cleft lip is swallowing when seen on ultrasound imaging. A static image or perceptible movement can be the result of this motion, it has to be judged by the difference in movement.

Diagnosing cleft lip using echotomography

Echotomography can accurately diagnose cleft lip, however the dynamic nature of this imaging approach may cause differences in the appearance of the cleft in each scan. Thus, a definitive diagnosis might require the use of several tests rather than depending on a single test. Minor forms of cleft lips and cleft palates, like incomplete clefts, may not be seen using echosonography.

Concerning genetic testing

When a condition is considered to have a hereditary foundation, genetic testing is used to determine the likelihood that an individual may get the disease or pass it on to siblings or others in the family. The genetic marker identification process is indispensably involved in the customization of preventive and therapeutic interventions. Blood samples are usually taken in order to examine relevant genes linked to the suspected congenital disorders. Genetic testing is widely used in Japan to diagnose diseases that are known to have hereditary roots, like hemophilia and muscular dystrophy. Cleft lip and palate are classified as a "multifactorial disease" due to their complicated interactions with both environmental and genetic factors. They are not currently included in standard genetic testing because the gene responsible for the condition has yet to be identified.

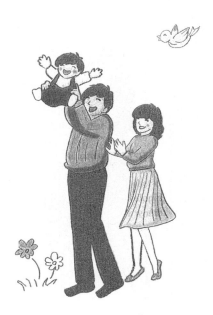

CHAPTER 1. BASIC INFORMATION ABOUT CLEFT LIP AND PALATE

Q 14. IS JAPANESE MEDICAL TREATMENT BEHIND OTHER COUNTRIES?

A Japanese healthcare is regarded as being among the best in the world.

Professional healthcare groups like the Japanese Cleft Palate Foundation concentrate exclusively on issues like cleft lip and palate in Japan. Annual professional conferences, both domestically and internationally, enhance the adoption of innovative treatment procedures by providing a forum for academics to share their experience. Because Japanese experts consistently collaborate with their international counterparts, such as the American Cleft Palate Craniofacial Association and the International Cleft Palate Foundation Japan's medical organizations have a global impact. In addition to publishing the findings of studies on Cleft lip and palate internationally, together with the International Cleft Palate Foundation hosts scholarly conferences in a number of nations each year to share latest information and technology. Japan is widely recognized for its skill in treating cleft lip and palate, leading many foreign countries to seek advice from Japanese experts, despite some parents choosing to seek treatment overseas.

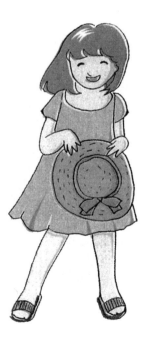

CHAPTER *2.* PRE-SURGERY AND SURGERY

CHAPTER 2. PRE-SURGERY AND SURGERY

Q 15. WHAT SHOULD BE PREPARED BEFORE SURGERY?

A It is recommended to prepare as follows:

Cleft lip surgery

This is done when the baby is 3-6 months old and weighs around 6 kg. Since the baby is not yet weaned, breastfeeding may be restricted for a few days post-surgery to allow the lip wound to heal. To prepare, practice feeding with a bottle (such as a pigeon-type bottle designed for cleft palate) or a spoon beforehand. For anesthesia management, the baby may be asked to drink sugar water before surgery. It's helpful to get them accustomed to this in advance. After the surgery, restraint tubes will be placed on both arms to prevent the baby from touching the wound. While these are usually provided by the hospital, you may also create your own (refer to a separate article for instructions).

Palatal surgery

This procedure is typically performed when the child is between 1.5 and 2 years old, weighing at least 10 kilograms, and after the first primary molar (the fourth tooth from the front) has fully erupted. After surgery, food is primarily taken orally. To reduce the risk of infection and promote healing, maintain good oral hygiene by brushing your child's teeth daily.

Revision, lip and palate reconstruction surgery, alveolar bone graft surgery and osteotomy surgery

These surgeries may be performed later to address functional or aesthetic concerns. For these procedures, oral hygiene is especially critical. Since these are performed at an age where the patient can care for their own mouth, develop a habit of brushing teeth after every meal and before bed well in advance of the surgery. Post-surgery, there may be temporary braces or intermaxillary fixation (where the jaw is wired shut). Follow the instructions provided by your doctor or dental hygienist closely. By preparing properly and following these guidelines, you can help ensure a smoother surgical process and recovery.

Q 16. EVEN AFTER SURGERY, WILL THE CLEFT LIP OR PALATE STILL BE NOTICEABLE?

A While the appearance significantly improves after about an hour of surgery, differences between the left and right sides may become more noticeable as you age. To address this, a nostril retainer is often used.

With advancements in surgery and technology, scars are almost invisible. However, immediately after surgery, the lips and nose achieve a beautiful, balanced shape. Over time, the difference between the left and right sides may become more noticeable due to postoperative scar contracture on the operated side and slower growth as you age. To anticipate this, surgeons often apply a technique called "overcorrection," leaving the left and right sides slightly asymmetrical right after surgery to account for future changes. To improve outcomes, wearing a nostril retainer is important. The specific method for wearing it may vary depending on the facility. For more details on nostril retainers, see the separate article Q34.

Q 17. PLEASE EXPLAIN THE TREATMENT AND SURGICAL PROCEDURES FOR CLEFT LIP AND PALATE FROM INFANCY TO ADULTHOOD

A Refer to the team approach outlined in the table 1.

Traditionally, treatment began after the child was born. However, with the remarkable advancements in prenatal diagnosis since 2010, cleft lip and palate can now be detected during pregnancy through methods such as ultrasound examination or even blood sampling from the mother.

Consequently, we are implementing strategies to prevent the occurrence of cleft lip and palate, which include genetic counseling before conception and interventions during pregnancy.

Counseling is provided, including the above.

The flow of treatment for cleft lip and palate patients is shown in the table below (Aichi Gakuin University Hospital). Treatment for cleft lip and palate does not end with oral surgery; it continues until adulthood. A team approach with a medical doctor, clinical psychologist, nurse, speech-language-hearing therapist, dietitian, dental hygienist, etc. are required.

CHAPTER 2. PRE-SURGERY AND SURGERY

Table 1. Multidisciplinary team approach for children with cleft lip and palate

Period	Treatment details	Clinical department
Before pregnancy	Genetic counseling	Oral Surgery
	Dietary advice on prevention of cleft lip and palate	Obstetrics and Gynecology
	Genetic testing	Pediatrics, Department of Nutrition
Prenatal (During pregnancy)	Counseling	Oral Surgery
		Obstetrics and Gynecology
		Pediatrics
		Clinical Psychologist
First examination	Hotz plate impression, nostril correction (nasal retainer), child development testing, counseling, Hotz plate fixing and management	Oral Surgery
	Feeding status	Speech Therapy Outpatient Clinic
	Inspection and assessment of the nasal retainer (Hotz plate with external nasal stent)	Oral Surgery
	Assessment of any complications	Pediatrics
	Nutrition control and management	Department of Nutrition
	Guidance for low birth weight infants are all included in the following: orientation, examination, breastfeeding, and guidance	Pediatrics
Approximately 6 months, 6 kg or more	Lip surgery (pre-operative examination, surgery, post-operative care)	Oral Surgery
		Pediatrics
		Anesthesiology
	Pre and Post-operative speech evaluation	Speech Therapy Outpatients Clinic
	Oral hygiene management	Pediatric Dentistry
	Otitis media examination and treatment	Otorhinolaryngology
1.5-2 years, 10 kg or more	Palatoplasty (pre-operative examination, surgery, post-operative care)	Oral Surgery
	(1st of 2 procedures) Mucosal flap, etc.	Pediatrics
		Anesthesiology
	Pre and Post-operative speech evaluation	Speech Therapy Outpatients Clinic
Around 4 years old and up	Speech and language development assessment and treatment (using nasopharyngeal fiber optics) (Speech Aid, Palatal Lift)	Speech Therapy Outpatient Clinic
	Lip and palate revision surgery (preoperative examination, surgery, postoperative care)	Oral Surgery
		Pediatrics, Internal Medicine
		Anesthesiology
	Pre and Post-operative speech and language evaluation	Speech Therapy Outpatients Clinic
Around 5 years old	Occlusion, Dental alignment examination and orthodontic treatment started, 2nd stage of two-stage palate repair palatal fistula closure*	Orthodontics

Ages 8-10 *Recently, it is often performed at the same time as upper jaw bone grafting	Alveolar bone grafting (foramen closure) surgery (preoperative examination, posoperative management), 2nd stage of two-stage palate repair palatal fistula closure*, Jaw correction (bone distraction method)	Oral Surgery, Pediatrics, Anesthesiology
	Pre and Post-operative speech and language evaluation	Speech Therapy Outpatient Clinic
	Occlusion, dentition, upper jaw development	Orthodontics
		Prosthodontics
		Department of Conservative Treatment
16 years old and over	Orthognathic surgery (pre-operative examination, surgery, post-operative management)	Oral Surgery
	Revision of labio nasal alar reconstruction (pre-operative examination, surgery, post-operative management)	Internal Medicine
		Anesthesiology
		Orthodontics
		Prosthodontics
		Department of Conservative Treatment
	Pre and Post-operative speech and language evaluation	Speech Therapy Outpatient Clinic

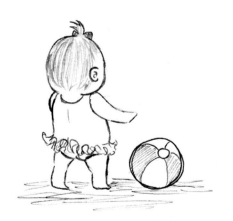

CHAPTER 2. PRE-SURGERY AND SURGERY

Q 18. CAN YOU EXPLAIN THE SURGICAL PROCEDURE FOR CLEFT LIP REPAIR?

A Please see below.

Timing of surgery for cleft lips

Due to nursing difficulties and the desire of the family to have the surgery as soon as feasible, several clinics used to perform cleft lip surgery right after birth. However, the majority of Japanese hospitals, including ours, now operate on babies weighing more than 6 kg between the ages of 3 and 5 months.

Surgery will be done in two stages if there are bilateral clefts, with a small gap of two to three months between each stage.

The reasons for this are:
① It is safer to give a newborn baby some time to adjust to its new surroundings because it has just left the mother's womb and is experiencing stress in a different natural setting. It's also possible that other issues won't be noticed right away after birth.
② Lip actions, such sucking, enhance the amount of the lip tissue, and surgery can complete morphogenesis. The orbicularis Oris muscle, which move the lips, are also developing at this period, which is beneficial for future lip motor function.
③ The technique is safer because anesthesia and subsequent care are simple.
④ There is not much of an impact on maxillary development.
⑤ Preoperative orthodontics, like that for the palate plate, can realign a misaligned jaw or nose, which eventually has a positive effect on the repair of deformities caused by surgery and etc. are possible.

We understand that families want the surgery to happen as soon as possible, but as was already indicated, it is preferable to wait a proper period of time when taking into account the baby's safety during the procedure and the outcome. So, please wait with patience for the positive benefit of a child.

Which tests are performed before to surgery?

Pre-operative testing

Before surgery, the attending physician, pediatrician, and anesthesiologist will perform a series of pre-operative tests to ensure your baby is in the best possible health for the procedure. These tests usually include a chest X-ray, urine analysis, and blood draws. While blood draws can seem intimidating, it's important to understand that newborns have less developed pain receptors than adults, and many babies may remain calm or even smile during the procedure. This suggests that the discomfort is not as severe as we might think. The primary goal of these tests is to confirm that your baby

22

is healthy and ready for surgery, minimizing any risks and maximizing the chances of a successful outcome.

In some cases, if the test results show any concerns, the surgery may need to be postponed. Additionally, if your baby develops a cold or shows any signs of illness before the scheduled surgery, it may also be delayed. While this can be disappointing for parents, especially if the illness seems minor, the decision to postpone is made with the baby's safety in mind. A team of specialists, including the lead physician, anesthesiologists, and nurses, will review the situation on the day of the surgery. If the baby is unwell, it's important to recognize that going ahead with surgery could increase the risk of complications, so the operation is rescheduled to ensure the best possible outcome for your baby.

Typically, mothers and babies are admitted to the hospital three days prior to surgery to allow time to adjust to the hospital environment and undergo any necessary pre-surgical testing. On the day before surgery, some babies may appear completely healthy, but in rare cases, a fever may develop. This is often a response to the stress and anxiety surrounding the surgery. It is important to remember that this is common and usually resolves once the surgery is postponed.

Cleft lip and palate surgery has advanced significantly, and when performed by a skilled specialist, the procedure is very safe. While it is natural for mothers to feel anxious as the surgery date approaches, it's equally important to remain calm. The medical team is highly experienced, and they will take every step to ensure the best care for your baby.

How is surgery for cleft lip done?

Parents often have many questions before cleft lip surgery, such as, "Does it hurt?" and "How long will the operation take?" It's natural for them to feel anxious, especially if they've never witnessed a surgical procedure before. Many parents turn to videos and online resources to understand what cleft lip surgery entails, which can sometimes lead to mixed emotions and uncertainty. To ease these concerns, here's a brief overview of what happens during the surgery at our institution.

Once the baby is brought into the operating room, they are gently placed on the operating table, and monitoring devices such as an electrocardiogram (ECG) and blood pressure monitor are attached to track their vital signs. Most babies appear puzzled at this stage, experiencing a new and slightly unusual sensation. Once the monitors are in place, the anesthesiologist uses a mask to administer a sweet-sour-smelling anesthetic gas to help the baby fall asleep. Initially, the mask is placed near, but not directly on, the baby's face to minimize discomfort or crying. After the baby is fully asleep, an intravenous (IV) line is inserted, which is completely painless as the baby is already unconscious. The anesthesiologist then inserts a breathing tube to deliver oxygen and anesthetic gas throughout the procedure. To protect the baby's eyes during surgery, eye drops are applied, and a small piece of tape is used for shielding.

Next, the surgical team, which includes the lead surgeon, two assisting surgeons, one or two anesthesiologists, and two nurses, begins preparing for the operation. The inside and outside of the baby's mouth are thoroughly cleaned, and the body is covered with a sterile drape called a compresence. The surgeon carefully maps out the procedure using a surgical tape measure and a special pen, ensuring absolute precision down to the millimeter. This preparation is meticulous and accounts for a signif-

CHAPTER 2. PRE-SURGERY AND SURGERY

icant portion of the surgical time. Various surgical techniques may be used, including the Millard method, the Cronin method, or adaptations of these approaches, depending on what is most suitable for the child. At our institution, we also employ a specialized method developed to optimize outcomes for our patients.

By sharing these steps, we hope to reassure parents about the care and precision involved in cleft lip surgery and to provide a clear understanding of what they can expect.

Once the surgical design for the cleft lip repair is completed, a hemostatic agent is injected into the lips to minimize bleeding, and the procedure begins after the medication takes effect. Cleft lip repair involves more than simply closing the cleft; it also includes reconstructing nasal deformities to restore symmetry and function, reapproximating the orbicularis Oris muscle to ensure proper lip movement, and, in some cases, performing adjunctive jaw procedures for babies with cleft palates to enhance the success of future surgeries. This comprehensive approach not only improves the aesthetic appearance but also supports better functional outcomes for feeding, speech, and overall oral development.

During cleft lip surgery, suturing is performed in multiple layers using specific needles and threads designed for each tissue type, such as skin, muscle, mucous membrane, and subcutaneous tissue. This meticulous approach ensures that the wound heals properly and significantly reduces the risk of reopening after surgery.

Once the procedure is complete, the anesthesiologist stops administering the anesthetic gas and switches to providing only oxygen to the baby's lungs. Protective tape covering the baby's eyes is carefully removed, and a nurse secures the IV line with a protective device to prevent it from being dislodged.

As the effects of the anesthetic gas wear off, the baby will gradually wake up on their own. When the baby is fully awake and responsive, the anesthesiologist removes the breathing tube from their mouth. The baby is then transferred to an observation room equipped with an oxygen tent, where their vital signs and overall health are closely monitored for a few hours.

Parents should be aware that the baby will not return to their hospital room immediately after surgery. This observation period is essential to ensure the baby's recovery is progressing smoothly and there are no complications. Some parents worry about the time it takes for their baby to wake up or the possibility of delays if the procedure takes longer than expected. However, these steps are crucial to provide a safe and effective recovery process for the baby. Rest assured that once the medical team confirms the baby's condition is stable, they will be returned to their hospital room to reunite with their family.

Things to consider after the surgery

① Transfer to the inpatient ward

After surgery, your baby will be transferred back to their hospital room wearing a cylindrical device called a restraint belt. This device is used to prevent your baby from touching or putting their hands near their mouth, which could interfere with the healing of the surgical site.

An intravenous (IV) drip will also be connected to your baby to provide essential fluids, nutrients, and any necessary medications. It's important to ensure the IV line stays secure, as replacing it can be challenging if your baby becomes agitated. To prevent accidental dislodgement, watch for any movements such as kicking or pulling at the IV tube. If the flow of the IV drip seems to stop or slow, please alert a nurse immediately for assistance.

Your baby may only be allowed to receive fluids when directed by the medical team. After surgery, the lingering effects of anesthesia may cause your baby to vomit, so fluid intake will be carefully monitored. While some parents worry about their baby not receiving milk for several hours before and after surgery, the IV drip ensures that all necessary fluids and nutrients are provided during this time.

Stitches will be removed approximately 4-9 days after surgery, depending on the surgical method used and the progress of wound healing. Please note that stitch removal is performed in the operating room, and delays may occur on weekends or holidays. Rest assured, the medical team will manage this process and provide updates as needed.

After surgery, it is common for babies to develop a mild fever. If necessary, the doctor will prescribe antipyretic medication to manage it. Secretions may also accumulate in your baby's throat due to the effects of general anesthesia. These secretions can sometimes make breathing difficult if they build up, so please notify a nurse immediately if you notice any signs of discomfort or labored breathing. Additionally, monitor your baby's urination. If there is little or no urine output, inform the nurse so the doctor can adjust the IV drip rate as needed.

On the first day after surgery, most babies tend to have low energy on the day of the surgery but typically regain their strength the following day. While the surgical wound may cause some initial discomfort, your baby may take slightly longer to drink milk. Please be patient and allow your baby time to feed adequately, as proper nutrition is essential for healing. The medical team will be there to support you and address any concerns throughout the recovery process.

After surgery, your baby will be provided with a special protective device, such as a tape protector or sponge padding, designed to shield the surgical wound from accidental impacts, such as when the baby rolls over. This device helps protect the healing tissue and ensures optimal recovery.

Some parents may request the same protective device that their other child used during a similar surgery. However, the choice of device is determined by the doctor based on the specific surgical technique used and the condition of the wound. The application of this protective device typically occurs a few days after the surgery, once the medical team evaluates the wound and confirms it is ready for additional support.

This individualized approach ensures that your baby receives the most appropriate care for their unique situation.

Seven to 10 days following surgery, patients are typically released from the hospital.

② **Hospital discharge**

After discharge, for about 2-3 months, we work to prevent scar formation by applying steroid ointment, covering the area with a cloth or special tape, and applying pressure with a Reston sponge. At this stage, however, the baby may remove the tape several times a day, which can be challenging for the family. Despite this, such home care significantly impacts the condition of the scar.

If necessary, a nasal retainer may also be inserted, taking into consideration the shape of the nostrils and nasal wings. Managing the nasal retainer requires a similar level of care and attention.

Jaw development

The reaction of the upper jaw to cleft lip surgery is primarily due to the impact on the upper jaw during the procedure. This reaction may occur because closing the cleft lip significantly increases lip pressure, which can affect the development and growth of the upper jaw.

Specialists are continually improving surgical techniques to minimize their impact on the upper jaw and carefully select the timing of the surgery to reduce potential complications. To monitor the upper jaw's development after surgery, regular X-rays of the head and impressions of the jaw are taken. If any issues with upper jaw growth are detected, appropriate treatment will be provided at the right time.

This is why regular follow-ups and health check-ups are essential after cleft lip or palate surgery. They allow healthcare providers to track your child's development and address any concerns early to ensure the best possible outcomes.

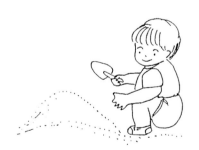

Q 19. PLEASE TELL ABOUT CLEFT PALATE SURGERY

A Please see below.

At many facilities, both the single-stage surgery method and the staged (two-step) surgery method are used, depending on the patient's needs and the surgical goals.

Timing of surgery

In Japan, cleft palate surgery is typically performed during the repetitive speech stage when a child begins to repeat sounds and words. This timing aims to support optimal speech development. At our facility, we prioritize achieving good speech outcomes while minimizing any impact on upper jaw (maxillary) development.

The surgery is usually scheduled when the baby is around 10 to 12 months old and weighs approximately 10 kilograms. However, the exact timing may vary depending on the child's overall health, growth, and any associated conditions.

A small percentage (approximately 5-10%) of children with cleft lip and palate have additional congenital anomalies. For these children, surgery may be delayed to address complications or stabilize their health.

In rare cases, a tissue deficit may result in a hole (fistula) forming in the anterior hard palate after surgery. Even if the fistula is significant, it can be effectively closed later using techniques such as a tongue flap. Parents should not worry about these possibilities, as they can be managed successfully.

Purpose of surgery

The primary goals of cleft palate surgery are:
1. **Functional Restoration**: To close the cleft and restore the function of the soft palate, enabling proper speech and swallowing.
2. **Nasopharyngeal Closure**: To separate the oral and nasal cavities, preventing nasal regurgitation and aiding in clear speech.
3. **Support Growth**: To minimize any interference with upper jaw development by carefully planning the surgery and postoperative care.

In the United States, some facilities perform cleft palate surgery as early as a few months after birth, while in Europe, surgery may be delayed to assess jaw growth. If there is significant underdevelopment of the upper jaw, orthodontic devices may be used before surgery to support jaw growth. The timing of surgery varies globally based on medical practices and the surgeon's evaluation of the child's needs.

Postoperative care

After cleft palate surgery, careful wound protection is essential. A protective device or bed may be

27

CHAPTER 2. PRE-SURGERY AND SURGERY

used to safeguard the surgical site. Post-surgery swelling and airway secretions may cause temporary difficulty breathing or swallowing. Nurses will assist in suctioning secretions to keep the airway clear.

Parents should note the following:

- **Dietary adjustments**: Initially, feeding may involve soft or liquid foods to avoid irritation to the surgical site.
- **Oral hygiene**: Post-surgery, proper oral care is crucial to prevent infections and ensure healing.
- **Hospital visits**: Regular follow-up visits will monitor healing and speech development.

Recently, some facilities in Japan have adopted single-stage surgery methods, reducing the need for multiple procedures. In cases requiring additional interventions, such as jaw surgeries or bone grafting, these are planned at a later stage based on the child's development.

By combining advanced surgical techniques with ongoing monitoring and therapy, we aim to ensure the best outcomes for both speech and upper jaw development in children with cleft palate.

After cleft palate surgery, it is important to encourage your child to gargle regularly to maintain good oral hygiene and reduce the risk of infection. The sutures used in the procedure are absorbable, so there is no need for removal.

Speech therapy

Most children will regain normal nasopharyngeal closure following surgery, which is necessary for proper separation between the oral and nasal cavities during speech and swallowing. However, some children may experience **hypernasality**, where air escapes through the nose while speaking, affecting speech clarity. In certain cases, children may maintain normal nasopharyngeal closure and not develop hypernasality.

Speech therapy is an important part of post-surgical care, as it helps children develop normal speech. At our facility, the Cleft Palate Center works closely with the Speech Therapy Outpatient Department to provide families with guidance on post-surgery speech training. The need for speech therapy and the timing of when to start it depend on the individual child's progress. Speech therapy is also available for children who have had surgery at other facilities, and if needed, we can refer you to a suitable facility in your area.

After surgery, some children may show a temporary tendency toward **palatalization**, which can cause speech errors as the mouth heals. Additionally, some children may experience bleeding from the surgical site, irregular teeth, or dental crowding. These issues are generally manageable with proper care and follow-up visits.

It is important for children to have regular speech evaluations to monitor their progress. At our facility, speech-language pathologists offer early orientation to parents, answering concerns and providing guidance on speech development. During the hospitalization period for cleft palate surgery, it is often possible to assess if further speech therapy or even secondary surgery may be necessary.

If the hospital where the initial surgery was performed does not have cleft palate specialists, continued monitoring and care for language development can be arranged at another specialized facility.

It is important to note that not all speech-language pathologists specialize in cleft palate care, so it is advisable to consult your doctor for a referral to a specialized facility near you.

For families residing near our hospital, specialized training by speech-language pathologists is also available. By maintaining regular follow-up visits and engaging in speech therapy, when necessary, children with cleft palates can achieve significant improvements in their speech and overall development.

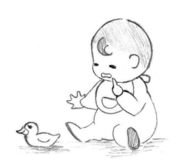

CHAPTER 2. PRE-SURGERY AND SURGERY

Q 20. WHY CAN'T SURGERY BE DONE IMMEDIATELY AFTER BIRTH?

A **The surgery can be performed immediately after birth; however, for safety reasons, it is generally considered more appropriate to perform the surgery at a later time, when it can yield better results.**

Cleft lip and palate surgery is usually performed shortly after birth, but the exact timing depends on several factors, including the baby's overall health and specific needs. The goal of the surgery is to close the cleft and ensure proper facial and oral development.

While it is possible that some complications may not be immediately apparent, the timing for surgery is generally determined by the child's weight and age. For cleft lip surgery, the procedure is typically performed when the baby reaches a weight of around 10 kg, which usually happens between 10 and 12 months of age. Similarly, cleft palate surgery is generally scheduled around this same weight milestone.

Although surgery is not performed immediately after birth, significant preoperative preparations can be made to improve the shape of the nose, narrow the cleft, and refine the nasal wings. These preparatory steps help achieve the best possible outcome. (**Fig. 1, 2**)

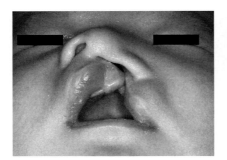   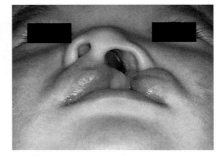

Fig. 1   At first examination   **Fig. 2   Just before surgery**

One of the advantages of performing surgery around this age is that the baby is generally more stable and prepared for the procedure, which can result in a quicker recovery. However, cleft lip and palate are not life-threatening conditions, so the surgery is not an emergency and can be planned accordingly.

It is also important to recognize that immediately after birth, babies are adjusting to a new environment and may be under some stress, which could lead to other health concerns. As such, while surgery is essential for improving the baby's quality of life, parents should be prepared to wait for the right moment to ensure the best possible outcome.

We understand that this waiting period can be stressful for parents, but it is important to remain patient and supportive as your child undergoes this critical stage of their treatment. Please trust that your medical team will work closely with you to ensure the best care and results for your baby.

Q 21. I HAVE BEEN TOLD THAT MY CHILD HAS A HEART CONDITION. CAN MY CHILD STILL HAVE SURGERY FOR CLEFT LIP AND PALATE?

A Yes, your child can undergo surgery for cleft lip and palate. While it may be scheduled later than the typical timing, the decision will be made after a thorough examination and considering the results.

Having a heart condition does not necessarily mean that surgery for cleft lip and palate is not possible. In fact, many children with cleft lip and palate also have heart conditions. Cardiologists, pediatricians, and anesthesiologists will perform detailed evaluations to assess the heart condition. If heart surgery is not required and the condition can be monitored, cleft lip and palate surgery can proceed at an appropriate time based on your child's health status.

If heart surgery is necessary before the cleft surgery, the heart surgery will be performed first, followed by the cleft lip and palate surgery once the heart condition has stabilized.

So, while surgery may be scheduled later than usual due to a heart condition, the timing and facility will be carefully determined based on your child's specific health needs and the examination results.

Q 22. HOW MANY SURGERIES ARE NEEDED FOR CLEFT LIP AND PALATE?

A There is no limit to the number of surgeries, but having too many is not a good idea.

There is no strict limit to the number of surgeries that can be performed for cleft lip and palate. However, it's important to note that while multiple surgeries are possible, the goal is to achieve the best possible outcome with the fewest surgeries. Too many surgeries are generally not beneficial, and it's preferable to focus on optimizing the results with each procedure. Additionally, after the second surgery, your child will still be eligible for health insurance and ongoing developmental medical care.

When surgery is repeated too many times, it can reduce the amount of available tissue and affect the development of the jaw. Some patients visit multiple hospitals to ensure safety, and with each surgery, cleft lip can become more challenging to treat. In these situations, it's important for parents to stay calm, carefully discuss the possibility of surgery with a specialist, and consider both the benefits and risks. There may be cases where parents or adult patients are dissatisfied with the outcome, face high medical costs, or experience speech difficulties due to scarring in the palate.

31

Q 23. PLEASE TELL ME ABOUT PREOPERATIVE CORRECTION FOR THE FIRST SURGERY

A It improves the shape of the alveolar ridge (the area of the jaw where the teeth will erupt), the maxilla (upper jaw), and the nose. The methods used for this include the Hotz plate, Nasoalveolar Molding (NAM), and Latham appliance. These preoperative treatments help to optimize the outcomes of surgery by guiding the growth and development of the oral and facial structures before the first surgery.

Hotz plate

The Hotz plate, also known as the artificial palate plate, helps improve the shape of the alveolar ridge and can make breastfeeding easier. Without intervention, the tongue may push into the cleft, causing the gap to widen and misalign the teeth. The plate helps improve the alveolar shape and supports proper breastfeeding by helping the tongue and palate work together more effectively.

NAM (Nasoalveolar molding) (Fig. 1)

NAM is used to improve the shape of the external nose and the dental arches. This method is common in many clinics and involves using an artificial plate that covers the mouth. The plate helps guide the growth of the upper jaw and supports the natural shape of the jaw. NAM also works to promote proper positioning of the teeth and improves the shape of the nose.

These orthodontic treatments are important steps in preparing for surgery and can improve both function and appearance, helping to achieve the best possible outcomes.

Before surgery, a device called Nasoalveolar Molding (NAM) is used to improve the external shape of the nose and the alignment of the jaw. NAM helps prepare the area for surgery by gently guiding

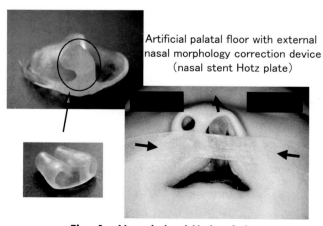

Fig. 1 Nasal stent Hotz plate

the growth of the jaw and nose. In cases of complete cleft lip, the nostrils are connected to the oral cavity, making it difficult to use a nostril retainer effectively. Instead, NAM uses a retainer attached to the jaw with a small metal pin, applying gentle pressure to reposition the jaw. This process is usually done under general anesthesia, though in some cases, local anesthesia may be used.

To enhance the effect, tape is often applied to keep the device in place and maximize its benefits. The NAM system also includes a device to correct the external nasal shape. While NAM and the **Latham appliance** are widely used in some facilities, fewer clinics may offer them.

In Japan, this treatment is sometimes referred to as an "artificial palate plate with external nasal morphology correction device." The goal of NAM is to help shape both the nasal and oral structures in preparation for the first surgery.

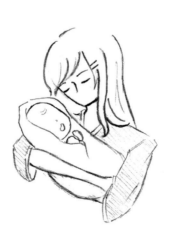

CHAPTER 2. PRE-SURGERY AND SURGERY

[Q] 24. CAN GENERAL ANESTHESIA CAUSE ANY OTHER PROBLEMS?

[A] General anesthesia, when administered by a trained anesthesiologist, is very safe and rarely causes problems.

There are two main types of anesthesia: general and local anesthesia. The key difference between the two is whether the patient is conscious during the procedure. With general anesthesia, the patient is made unconscious, which means they cannot feel pain or communicate during the surgery. Throughout the procedure, the anesthesiologist closely monitors the patient's condition to ensure there are no complications.

General anesthesia is used safely across a wide range of ages, from infants to adults, and advances in medical technology have made it even safer. The skills of anesthesiologists have also improved, meaning that the risks of anesthesia are very low, even in children. In fact, while anesthesia-related accidents do happen, the chances are much lower than the risk of fatal traffic accidents.

For children, general anesthesia is often chosen for even minor procedures because children cannot stay still during surgery, and it helps avoid the emotional distress of being awake. The use of general anesthesia ensures the child's safety during the procedure.

Various medications are used in general anesthesia, and the right drugs are carefully chosen based on the patient's specific needs to minimize the risk of complications. Some side effects may run in families, so a thorough pre-surgery consultation with the anesthesiologist is important.

While it's true that frequent procedures like surgery and anesthesia may not directly impact a child's psychological health, the emotional impact of surgery and anesthesia is something everyone, including doctors, nurses, and family, must be aware of and manage carefully to help reduce anxiety for the child.

If you have any concerns about anesthesia, it's a good idea to speak with both the surgeon and the anesthesiologist.

34

Q 25. WHAT ARE THE EFFECTS OF X-RAYS TAKEN FOR THE TREATMENT OF CLEFT LIP AND PALATE ON THE BODY?

A The amount of radiation used during normal X-ray imaging is very small and does not cause any noticeable physical symptoms.

X-ray examinations use radiation (X-rays), which can have effects on the human body. However, they are essential for diagnosing conditions and guiding treatment. It's important to understand that the radiation from X-rays used for imaging is not harmful in the amounts typically used during these exams.

The effects of X-rays on the body depend on the area being exposed, and problems can occur if too much radiation is used, known as the "threshold dose." However, the radiation from standard X-ray imaging is much lower than this threshold, so no physical symptoms occur.

Since cleft lip and palate treatments are often done on young children, it's good to know that children are less sensitive to radiation than adults. The radiation dose required for children's X-rays is also lower, so there's no need to worry about harmful effects from the imaging.

Although children will likely need X-ray exams during their treatment, studies have not shown any harmful effects from the radiation used. The X-ray equipment is designed to target only the area that needs to be examined. There is also some scatter radiation (similar to how water sprays from a faucet), but this is much smaller compared to the direct radiation dose. Protective clothing is used during exams to further minimize exposure.

You can safely assist your child during the exam, as there's no risk to you from being in the room with them. The goal is to use the minimum necessary radiation to get an accurate diagnosis. Therefore, you can feel confident about the safety of the X-ray examination.

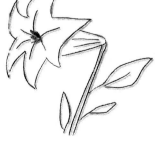

CHAPTER 2. PRE-SURGERY AND SURGERY

[Q] 26. CAN I BORROW X-RAYS AND TEST RESULTS FROM THE FACILITY I AM CURRENTLY VISITING WHEN GETTING A SECOND OPINION AT ANOTHER FACILITY?

[A] **Yes, getting a second opinion is your right as a patient. You can ask your current doctor for your X-rays and test results so you can share them with the doctor providing the second opinion.**

A second opinion means consulting another doctor to get their perspective on your child's treatment plan. This has become a more common practice because healthcare today involves patients in making decisions about their treatment, after being fully informed and giving consent (informed consent). A second opinion does not necessarily mean changing doctors, but rather, seeking advice from another doctor while continuing to work with your current primary care physician.

Some parents may feel concerned about asking for a second opinion, fearing it might harm their relationship with the doctor. However, a second opinion is about working together with your primary care doctor to choose the best treatment plan for your child. In most cases, there is no need to worry. It's important to remember that some doctors might not fully understand or support the idea of a second opinion, and they may suggest transferring care to another hospital or doctor. In such cases, you should carefully evaluate whether you feel comfortable continuing care with that doctor.

When seeking a second opinion, it's important to know what you want to achieve. If you ask simply whether the first opinion is correct, the answer will likely be "yes," unless there's a major issue. To get the most out of a second opinion, organize your thoughts and decide what you want to understand better before approaching another doctor.

Before seeking a second opinion, talk to your current doctor. Ask them to provide a medical record with all the necessary information for the new doctor to review. This will help the second doctor understand your child's history and treatment so they can offer the best advice.

Keep in mind that a second opinion is considered a consultation, not a treatment. Since it's not covered by health insurance, you will need to pay for the consultation yourself.

[Q] 27. HOW TO HELP YOUR CHILD GAIN WEIGHT BEFORE PALATE SURGERY

[A] Above all, try not to disturb your daily routine.

It's important to maintain a regular daily routine as your child prepares for palate surgery. At around 20 months of age, your child will start to develop a better balance between sleep, eating, and play. By providing three balanced meals each day on a regular schedule, your child will begin to feel hungry at the right times and eat properly.

When your child is about to have cleft palate surgery, avoid giving them their favorite foods or sweets just because they aren't eating enough. While it's important not to force them to eat, giving only their favorite foods may make it harder for them to return to a normal eating routine after surgery.

Since three meals a day may not provide enough of the necessary nutrients (like energy and protein), it's a good idea to offer snacks in addition to meals.

These snacks should be given after they have already eaten their three meals.

Some examples of healthy snacks include protein-rich foods like eggs, cheese, or meat, and calcium-rich foods like dairy products or leafy greens. You can also offer healthy snacks like fruits, yogurt, or nuts.

Important note: Snacks don't just mean sugary treats like biscuits or crackers. Focus on snacks that provide essential nutrients, especially those that support your child's growth and help with weight gain.

Children often need to gain some extra weight before surgery, so it's crucial to stick to a regular eating schedule. Even if your child is reluctant to eat, try not to disrupt their daily rhythm by constantly offering snacks or sweets.

If your child is around 12 months old, you may also consider switching to cow's milk, but be mindful of their preferences. If your child refuses cow's milk, you may need to get creative with how you incorporate it into their diet.

Common causes of poor weight gain:
- Unbalanced eating habits
- Too few or too many food options
- Individual constitution or preferences

Remember, children have smaller bodies and smaller stomachs than adults, so they can eat less at each meal. To make sure they get enough energy, consider offering drinks with energy as part of their daily intake. However, be careful not to give too many snacks, as this can affect their appetite for main meals.

Gradually introduce new foods by mixing them together—try combining rice balls, mashed potatoes, fruits, and dairy products. This way, your child can get used to new textures and tastes while still ensuring they gain the weight needed for surgery.

Importance of fats in your child's diet

When preparing baby food or infant food, many parents are unsure about the role of fats in their child's diet. Some may say things like, "I don't want to give them too much," "They shouldn't have fats," or "I'm not sure how much to use." While it's important not to overuse fats, including the right amount can expand the range of foods you can prepare and help your child get the nutrients they need.

Fats are one of the three major nutrients, along with carbohydrates and proteins. They are essential for your child's health. Fats provide energy, help build cell membranes, and are important for making hormones. Fats also help with the absorption of fat-soluble vitamins like A, D, E, and K. If your child doesn't get enough fat, their energy levels, immune system, and ability to fight infections may be affected.

If you haven't used fats in your child's meals yet, you can start by adding a small amount of butter to cooked vegetables or mixing in a bit of oil. This way, your child can get used to the taste of healthy fats without overdoing it.

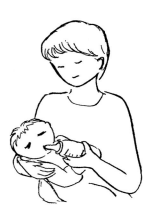

Q 28. MY CHILD SUCKS THEIR THUMB. HOW CAN WE ADDRESS THIS BEFORE SURGERY?

A There is nothing wrong with thumb sucking, but you should be aware of the following points:

Thumb sucking is a normal behavior, and it doesn't cause harm to your child, even if they are about to have cleft lip and palate surgery. Thumb sucking is a natural part of infant development, and it helps babies recognize their hands as part of their own body. It's very common for babies to suck their thumbs, and this behavior may continue for several months.

Cleft lip surgery often performs between 3-6 months of age. This coincides with the time when children start sucking their thumbs. After cleft lip surgery, it's important to avoid the child touching the surgical wound to prevent infection or complications. In the first 7-10 days after surgery, the stitches will need to heal, so a device may be used to keep your child from sucking their thumb or touching the area. Sometimes, children will continue thumb sucking into toddlerhood, but this can cause issues like misaligned teeth or bite problems. If thumb sucking continues past the age of 2 years, it may affect your child's dental development, so it's important to monitor the behavior closely.

A device may be used after surgery to prevent thumb sucking from interfering with the healing process. Thumb sucking is a common behavior that usually calms down by 10-15 months of age, but in some cases, it may persist longer. It's important to ensure your child doesn't continue this behavior for too long, as it can have negative effects on both their health and healing after surgery.

It is important to encourage awareness and provide support from those around. If a child undergoes lip or nose correction surgery before entering school, the surgery may be the trigger for the child to stop sucking their thumb.

CHAPTER 2. PRE-SURGERY AND SURGERY

[Q] 29. WHY IS VACCINATION BEFORE CLEFT LIP AND PALATE SURGERY RESTRICTED, AND HOW SHOULD POST-SURGERY VACCINATIONS BE MANAGED?

[A] **Side effects from vaccinations and complications during surgery, though rare, are not completely eliminated. In cases where there is no urgent need, such as with cleft lip and palate surgery, it is important to minimize any potential risks caused by recent vaccinations. Additionally, the general recommendation is to wait at least two weeks after surgery before administering any vaccinations. However, the timing of vaccinations will be determined based on each child's developmental progress and current health condition.**

Before surgery for cleft lip and palate, it's important to plan vaccinations carefully. Vaccinations should generally not be given right before surgery for a few reasons. First, there can be side effects from vaccines, and these side effects may overlap with the recovery process from surgery. Additionally, while surgery itself carries some risks, we want to minimize the risk of any "mixed-in" effects that could complicate the healing process, such as a reaction to a recent vaccination.

The best time to give vaccinations is typically **2 weeks after surgery**, but the exact timing will depend on your child's development and health condition. It is essential to ensure that vaccinations do not interfere with the surgical recovery process, as the body needs to focus on healing from the procedure.

In Japan, vaccination schedules have become crowded, with several vaccinations often scheduled at the same time. This can sometimes overlap with the timing of surgery. For this reason, it's important to avoid getting vaccinations too close to surgery to reduce the chances of complications.

However, vaccinations are crucial, and **prevention is better than cure**. If there is an urgent need for a vaccine due to an outbreak of disease in your area or a high-risk situation, a healthcare professional will guide you on the best course of action.

When scheduling your child's cleft lip and palate surgery, talk to the doctor about your child's vaccination schedule. Your doctor will help ensure that the timing of both surgery and vaccinations works together to avoid complications.

How long before surgery should vaccinations be given?

The timing of vaccinations before surgery depends on the type of vaccine. Some vaccines may need to be given several weeks before surgery, while others can be administered after the surgery, depending on the child's health and the urgency of the situation. It's always best to follow the guidance of your healthcare provider for the specific needs of your child.

40

When should vaccines be given after surgery?

Live vaccines: It's generally recommended to wait at least 2 weeks (or more) after surgery before administering live vaccines, such as the measles, mumps, and rubella (MMR) vaccine.

Inactivated vaccines and toxoids: These vaccines typically require a waiting period of 3 weeks (or more) after surgery, but the timing may vary depending on your child's overall health and recovery.

The reason for these waiting periods is that after surgery, the body needs time to heal. Vaccinations can cause side effects like fever or a rash, which may interfere with your child's recovery. Even vaccines such as the live polio vaccine can cause side effects quickly, often within hours, so it's important to plan vaccinations carefully to avoid complications.

Recovering from surgery can be very stressful for infants and young children. Therefore, it's important to consult with your child's pediatrician before scheduling any vaccinations after surgery. The timing of vaccines will depend on your child's recovery progress, health condition, and individual needs.

The standard practice is to wait 4 weeks after surgery. It's also important to note that while vaccines are essential for disease prevention, the timing of vaccinations needs to be carefully managed, especially around surgery, to ensure your child's well-being.

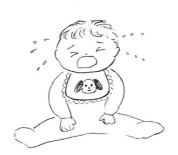

CHAPTER 2. PRE-SURGERY AND SURGERY

Q 30. WHEN HOSPITALIZED, IS IT BETTER TO HAVE A PRIVATE ROOM OR A SHARED ROOM?

A It is difficult to say which is better in general.

When deciding between a private room or a shared room during hospitalization, both options have their pros and cons, and the best choice depends on your preferences and the hospital's policies.

A private room offers more privacy and comfort, as it gives you the freedom to care for your child without the presence of others. It also provides a quiet space, which can be helpful for rest. However, private rooms are usually more expensive, and the cost is often not covered by insurance unless under special circumstances. It also allows for more space, which can make it easier for parents to stay with their child.

In a shared room, you will be with other families, which can be beneficial in certain ways. For example, you may have the opportunity to talk to other parents, especially mothers, who are going through similar experiences. This can provide emotional support and the chance to share tips and advice. Some parents form lasting friendships with other families they meet in shared rooms, and children may interact with each other, which can be positive for social development. However, shared rooms can be less private and sometimes less comfortable.

Ultimately, the decision depends on your priorities: whether you value privacy and comfort or the opportunity for support and interaction with other families. It's important to consider your child's needs, as well as your own, when making this decision.

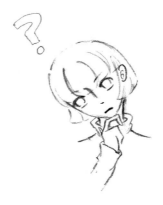

42

Q 31. FREQUENTLY ASKED QUESTIONS: ARM RESTRAINTS

A Below are some typical questions:

What are arm restraints?

Arm restraints are devices designed to prevent a child from engaging in behaviors such as thumb sucking or putting toys in their mouth after surgery, particularly when they have a cleft lip or palate repair.

The main purpose of the restraint is to keep the surgical site protected and prevent the child from touching the wound, which could cause irritation or disrupt healing. This helps avoid any contact with the healing area, ensuring that the surgical site remains undisturbed.

Restraints are especially useful during the early stages of recovery when the child may not understand the importance of keeping the area clean and intact. Typically, restraints are used until the stitches are removed and the surgical site is sufficiently healed. After the stitches are removed, the tissue from the surgery will be attached securely, and it will be less likely for the wound to open.

However, it's important to avoid direct contact with the wound even after the stitches are removed, so tape may be used to protect it during recovery.

How long should arms restraints be used after surgery?

The use of restraint is generally required until the stitches are removed and the wound has started to heal. Once the stitches are removed, the risk of the wound reopening is minimal, but it's still important to avoid touching the area. Restraints can be removed once the risk of disruption is low around 7-10 days after surgery, but this decision should always be made with guidance from the medical team.

Should a child practice wearing restraint at home?

There is no need to practice wearing restraint at home. While restraints are necessary for the safety and recovery of the child, they can be physically and emotionally stressful for young children, especially those who may not fully understand why they are being used. It's best to minimize their use whenever possible, and they should only be applied when necessary for treatment, with care and attention from parents.

In summary, arm restraints help prevent harmful contact with the surgical site, ensuring proper healing. However, they should be used only for the required period, and the child's comfort and well-being should always be prioritized.

43

CHAPTER 2. PRE-SURGERY AND SURGERY

[Q] 32. IT HAS BEEN A MONTH SINCE MY CLEFT LIP SURGERY, BUT THE REDNESS OF MY SCARS HAS NOT FADED, AND I STILL HAVE VISIBLE SCARS. WHAT SHOULD I DO?

[A] **After cleft surgery, it is common for parents to notice some redness at the surgical site or a hardening of the area around the wound. These symptoms are a normal part of the healing process and typically improve within 6 to 12 months after surgery. However, recovery times may vary depending on the individual.**

In rare cases, if there is no improvement within this time frame, the condition may develop into a keloid. A keloid is a type of thick, raised scar that can occur when the body produces excessive scar tissue during healing. To prevent or manage the development of keloids, some medical facilities may recommend:

- **Tranilast:** A medication that helps reduce excessive scar formation.
- **Steroid applications:** Steroid creams or injections to minimize inflammation and control scar tissue growth.
- **Pressure therapy:** Applying special tape to the area to provide gentle pressure, which can help reduce the risk of keloid formation.

These treatments are typically tailored to each child's needs and are carefully monitored by the medical team.

Q 33. PLEASE TELL ME HOW TO FEED MY CHILD AFTER CLEFT LIP SURGERY

A You can generally continue using the same bottle as before the surgery. However, if your child seems uncomfortable due to the bottle touching the surgical site, consider using a dropper to gently place milk at the back of their mouth. This can help avoid irritation to the wound while ensuring proper feeding.

Pigeon's narrow-mouthed bottle may be effective. It is possible to feed your baby directly from the mother's breast. However, if the nipple touches the wound after surgery due to swelling, etc., and the baby seems to dislike feeding, try using a long, thin bottle like a dropper (**Fig. 1**), so you can feed your baby without touching the wound after cleft lip surgery. This is a good idea in such cases, but it is not recommended until the stitches are removed, as it will touch a wide area of the wound.

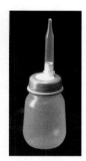

Fig. 1   Narrow-mouthed bottle

Q 34. WHAT EFFECT DOES A RETAINER NOSTRIL HAVE?

A After surgery or trauma, scarring around the nostrils and reduced elasticity of the surrounding tissue can cause deformities that narrow the nostrils. A retainer nostril is designed to help prevent this deformation by maintaining the nostrils' shape and suppressing narrowing.

When the body experiences an injury, whether from surgery or trauma, scar tissue forms as part of the healing process. During this process, scars may contract, pulling the surrounding tissues and leading to deformation around the affected area. Additionally, if surgery alters the shape of a structure, the natural elasticity of the surrounding tissues may cause it to return to its previous shape, a phenomenon known as tissue recoil.

This process also applies to the nostrils. After cleft-related surgery, the scars that form around the nostrils, combined with the elasticity of the surrounding tissues, can lead to narrowing or other deformations of the nostrils.

CHAPTER 2. PRE-SURGERY AND SURGERY

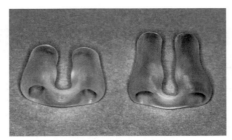

Fig. 1 Nasal retainer

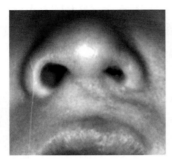   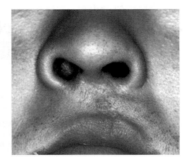

Fig. 2 Before using Nasal retainer   Fig. 3 After using Nasal retainer for 12 years

To manage and prevent such deformation, nasal retainers are often used. These devices help maintain the desired shape by counteracting the effects of scar contraction and tissue recoil.

(**Fig. 1**) illustrates nasal retainer, whereas (**Fig. 2**) shows narrowed nostrils (stenosis). In some facilities, it is used until the child's growth has stabilized. The product is typically used for a period ranging from 6 months to 1-year post-surgery.

In cases of nostril stenosis (**Fig. 3**), it is also utilized over an extended period during the growth phase to suppress deformation and guide proper correct development.

Wearing the product consistently for a long duration may lead to significant improvement in the condition mentioned above.

Q 35. WHY IS A PROTECTIVE PLATE USED AFTER CLEFT PALATE SURGERY?

A It helps protect the scar after surgery as it heals and prevents the upper jaw (maxilla) from becoming too narrow, supporting your child's healthy growth and development.

After cleft palate surgery, it's important to know that, unlike other parts of the body, the wound inside the mouth cannot be covered with bandages or tape. Instead, a special device called a protective plate is used (**Fig. 1**).

The protective plate plays a key role in stopping bleeding from the wound right after surgery and protecting the area while it heals. However, there is something important to remember: you must remove the plate regularly to clean both the plate and your child's teeth. If you don't, cavities can easily develop, which could affect your child's oral health.

For about three months after the surgery (**Fig. 2**), extra care is needed during the healing process. As the wound heals, the scar tissue can shrink (a process called scar contraction), which may cause the upper jaw (maxilla) to become narrower. This narrowing can affect your child's jaw development. So, keeping the mouth clean and using the protective plate correctly are essential to ensure successful healing and to prevent complications like cavities or jaw narrowing.

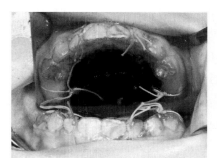

Fig. 1　Protective floor used immediately after surgery

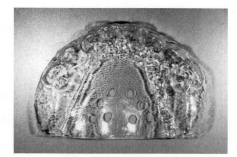

Fig. 2　Protective floor to be used from discharge until 3 months after surgery

CHAPTER 2. PRE-SURGERY AND SURGERY

[Q] 36. WHAT PRECAUTIONS SHOULD PARENTS TAKE AFTER THE CHILD IS DISCHARGED?

[A] **After cleft lip surgery, follow the doctor's instructions carefully. Avoid exposing the surgical site to direct sunlight for long periods of time for 6 months, and use sunscreen if your child is outdoors. Ensure that nasal retainer is used as instructed to support proper healing. After cleft palate surgery, keep the protective sheet or plate in place at all times during the first month to prevent bleeding and protect the wound. Feed your child soft foods during this period to avoid putting strain on the surgical site.**

For both cleft lip and palate surgeries, the frequency of hospital visits will depend on the wound's condition. Generally, during the 1st month, you should visit the hospital about once every two weeks and about once a month for the first six months after surgery.

After cleft lip surgery, your child will be discharged once the stitches are removed and there are no issues with the wound. Post-discharge, the nose will be supported by the nasal retainer with pressure for an extended period to help shape it properly. If the pressure on nose is too strong, surrounding areas may become red. In this case, please consult with your doctor.

To minimize the appearance of the lip scar, your doctor may recommend using steroid-containing tape or ointment on the wound, along with oral medication. Protecting the area from direct sunlight is essential, as the skin is more prone to absorbing ultraviolet rays, which can lead to melanin pigmentation. Sunscreen should be applied regularly when outdoors. Initially, the wound may appear red, but this is normal, and it is safe to wash or gently wipe the area during baths in the first week to month after surgery. For the first six months, hospital visits will typically occur about once a month to monitor healing and address any concerns. During this time, it is crucial to avoid prolonged exposure to direct sunlight and protect child's lip/upper jaw from pressure or strain to ensure proper recovery. Consult your doctor if you have any specific questions or concerns about the healing process.

After cleft palate surgery, it is safest to use a protective plate (wound protector) to shield the surgical site. With the protective plate in place, bleeding from the wound is minimal. However, food particles can accumulate on the protective plate, making the wound sensitive. To address this, brush only the front part of the upper palate and encourage your child to drink tea after meals to help prevent food from staying on the wound. This also supports the practice of improving the movement of the soft palate, which is essential for proper healing and function.

The frequency of hospital visits will depend on the condition of the wound, but you will be discharged once the initial healing is stable. Be aware that there is a small risk of postoperative infection. For the first month after surgery, the protective bed should remain in place at all times to minimize the risk of bleeding. However, after meals, remove the protective bed, wash it thoroughly, and then replace it. During this time, ensure your child eats only soft foods to reduce strain on the wound.

Since the protective bed can easily become unhygienic, brushing your child's teeth thoroughly is essential. Initially, you may feel hesitant to touch the wound, but gentle care is important. Gradually, you can begin brushing the back of the upper palate as well. After two months, the wound will have stabilized, and your child can start practicing activities like blowing and sucking using straws, flutes, or harmonicas to strengthen soft palate movement. Blowing involves continuous exhaling and sucking motions, which help improve oral function.

For the first six months after surgery, hospital visits will typically occur about once every two weeks, and for the following months once a month to monitor healing and progress. These steps will help support your child's recovery and overall oral health.

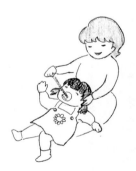

37. WHAT IS VESTIBULOPLASTY, AND WHY IS IT PERFORMED?

A This is a surgery to widen the oral vestibule.

This surgery, called oral vestibuloplasty, is performed to widen the oral vestibule. The oral vestibule is the space between the gums and lips at the front of the mouth. After cheiloplasty (lip repair surgery), this area may remain shallow due to limited soft tissue. In severe cases, this can lead to the lips forming a periodontal pocket, which can cause dental plaque and cause oral health issues.

For children with a cleft lip, tissue from the gums may have been transferred to the lips during previous surgery, particularly near the cleft's edge. This transferred tissue might even connect directly to the mucous membrane in the area that corresponds to the oral vestibule. In such cases, the lips may appear closed or constricted, limiting function and making this surgery necessary to improve oral structure and health.

Children with clefts may experience difficulty playing instruments like the flute or may face challenges with orthodontic treatments due to a shallow or narrow oral vestibule. To improve these issues, a surgery called vestibular reconstruction may be performed to create more space in the oral vestibule.

Even if the condition is not severe, having a shallow oral vestibule can make it difficult for your child to brush their teeth properly. In such situations, a surgical incision may be made in the narrow area to widen the vestibule and allow the tissue to flow, making oral care and speech functions easier. (**Fig. 1**, **Fig. 2**)

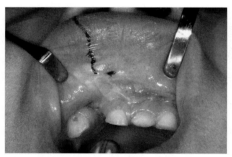
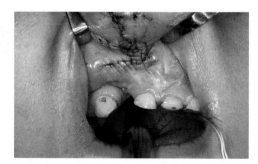

Fig. 1 Before oral vestibuloplasty   Fig. 2 Post-oral vestibuloplasty

[Q] 38. WHEN IS REVISION SURGERY FOR CLEFT LIP OR PALATE NECESSARY?

[A] The timing of surgery varies.

While it is best to minimize the number of surgeries, revision surgery may be needed for children with clefts based on several factors. These include the size of the cleft, the position of the mid-jaw (front teeth of the upper jaw), and how the cleft affects the child's social life and overall well-being.

In some cases, nasal deformities can occur, leading to issues such as the displacement or deformity of the alar cartilage (the cartilage around the nostrils), upper jawbone problems, and nasal septum misalignment. Scarring and displacement of the alar cartilage may also happen, depending on the child's specific condition.

Children may also experience **lip deformities**, which can affect the symmetry of the lips, the alignment of the lip line (vermilion), and the shape and thickness of the lips themselves. These issues are often caused by the natural growth process and can result in facial asymmetry, scarring, or underdevelopment of the upper jaw.

Even with corrective surgery performed at a young age, nasal deformities may reappear as the child grows. This is why, at our facility, we typically perform revision surgery to address nasal deformities after the age of 16, as the child's facial structures are more developed. In cases of significant nasal deformity, corrective surgery may be needed to improve the appearance and function of the nose and lips.

If parents are concerned about their child's **upper jaw (maxilla) deformity**, it is important to understand that we avoid performing surgical orthodontics at a young age, as it is typically not recommended. Instead, we use techniques like maxillary protraction (a process to help move the upper jaw forward) to improve jaw alignment before considering surgery around 4 years old as needed.

Once the child's jaw growth is complete, usually around the age of 16, we may perform osteotomy surgery, which can involve both the upper and lower jaws. This surgery is done in consultation with an orthodontist and prosthodontic specialist to ensure the best outcome for your child's jaw alignment and overall facial structure.

CHAPTER 2. PRE-SURGERY AND SURGERY

[Q] 39. WHAT TREATMENTS ARE AVAILABLE FOR PRESCHOOL AND SCHOOL-AGE CHILDREN?

[A] **It depends on the age and type of cleft, so please consult with a specialist.**

The purpose of regular check-ups

The schedule for regular checkups is set, and it may feel like most of the treatment for cleft lip and palate has already been completed by this stage. For some families, it might seem inconvenient to travel a long distance and wait for an extended time only to have a photograph taken, with the actual examination lasting just a short while. However, the primary purpose of regular checkups is to detect and address any new or ongoing issues that may require treatment at this stage. For families of children with cleft lip and palate, early childhood and school age are typically when the primary surgeries have been completed, and the children are mentally more stable compared to the period before surgery. Regular checkups often include procedures such as taking jaw impressions or, X-rays. Because of this, some parents may be tempted to skip these visits. Nevertheless, this stage is critical, as children may still experience challenges such as speech difficulties, ear infections, narrowing of the maxilla or dental arch, or concerns related to appearance. Regular checkups are essential for identifying and managing these issues effectively. The need for treatment and the timing of its initiation depends on the individual condition of each child. Regular checkups are essential to ensure that any necessary treatment is initiated at the most appropriate time.

Surgical interventions and timing

For cleft lip, primary cleft lip surgery is typically performed at around 3 months to 4 months of age after birth can produce significant results. However, deformation and scarring may occur, especially in the surgical wound. If there is excessive scarring or misalignment of the red lip border as time passes, it is recommended that parents wait until the child starts school (around age 5), taking into consideration the child's social life.

However, for nasal deformities, we do not perform extensive surgery such as inserting artificial materials, correcting the nasal alar cartilage, or upper jaw correction (correcting misalignment of the teeth through surgery). This is because even if correction is made at a young age, distortions will occur as the child grows.

For cleft palate, primary cleft palate surgery is performed around 18 months of age, after which from around 2 years of age, training is conducted to improve the ability of the muscles involved in the velopharyngeal closure function, such as levator veli palatini and palatopharyngeal muscles, through straw-blowing etc. Generally, about 55% of children with cleft palate naturally acquire velopharyngeal closure function with this simple training and are able to speak normal language, but the

52

remaining 15% of children will develop a nasalance due to nasal leakage of nasal air, and will require speech treatment from a speech- language therapist. Secondary surgeries, such as insufflation pharyngoplasty, pharyngeal flap reconstruction, and revision palatoplasty, may be performed at an appropriate stage based on the patient's needs.

Alveolar bone grafting

Bone grafting may also be performed in the cleft region of the palate to support the eruption of permanent teeth, such as canines, and to facilitate proper alignment of teeth through orthodontics, typically at around 7-12 years old.

Transplant materials for these surgeries often include the patient's own bone for optimal outcomes. Common donor sites are the ilium (hip bone), although in recent years, the mandible (lower jaw) and tibia (shinbone) have also been used as sources for bone grafts.

Orthodontic treatment, including the use of expansion plates and alignment of teeth, is often initiated during childhood or adolescence. The timing and materials used in these treatments are highly individualized, requiring careful consultation with doctors and orthodontists.

Parents are encouraged to seek second opinions and consult organizations like the Japanese Cleft Palate Foundation, which provide support and information for managing complex cases. Early correction of speech issues and promoting dental health are priorities to ensure the child's long-term well-being and social integration.

Contact information:

Japanese Cleft Palate Foundation

Tel: 052-757-4312

Hours: Monday to Friday, 10:00 AM — 4:00 PM

Cleft palate: Otitis media and orthodontic treatment

It is well-documented that individuals with a cleft palate are more susceptible to otitis media. This increased risk is due to the congenital hypoplasia of the levator veli palatini muscle, located near the oral side of the Eustachian tube (the tube connecting the ear to the mouth). The abnormal development of this muscle, often associated with cleft palate, impairs the normal functioning of the Eustachian tube.

Parents often wonder whether their child's teeth will grow in properly. In most cases, teeth develop normally, except in the cleft area. Artificial teeth can be placed in the cleft region after waiting for the jaw to mature. While parents are often thrilled to see their child's, teeth develop during toddler and school years, significant cavities may prevent the use of orthodontic devices to realign teeth. To prepare for potential orthodontic treatment, it is vital to establish good oral hygiene habits early. Since orthodontic appliances increase the risk of plaque accumulation, parents should assist their children with brushing their teeth until they are capable of doing so effectively on their own, typically around the age when they can wash their own hair. Additionally, parents should familiarize themselves with foods that contribute to cavities versus those that do not, particularly when providing snacks.

Orthodontic treatment has become increasingly common, yet cavities remain a concern due to

CHAPTER 2. PRE-SURGERY AND SURGERY

factors such as gingivitis and insufficient oral hygiene. The timing of orthodontic treatment varies for each child and should be decided by a team of specialists, including an orthodontist, oral surgeon, and speech therapist. In cases where jaw underdevelopment or palate abnormalities significantly impact speech, treatment may begin as early as infancy. However, most orthodontic treatments typically commence around age 12. During orthodontic treatment, removable appliances should be taken out after meals, and the teeth and appliances should be cleaned thoroughly to prevent food particles from causing cavities or staining.

It is crucial for children with cleft lip and palate to have access to dental specialists experienced in managing their unique needs. Children with cleft palates experience some degree of abnormal teeth alignment, underscoring the importance of regular specialist care. Parents should supervise their children's brushing to ensure no areas are left uncleaned, as this can significantly improve oral health and prevent cavities.

Preventing dental caries is especially important for children with cleft lip and palate. Dentists can provide valuable advice on proper brushing techniques and fluoride application to strengthen teeth. Misaligned teeth or an underdeveloped jaw can also negatively affect speech, making regular dental and hearing checkups essential. Furthermore, combining dental care with hearing evaluations is recommended, as children with cleft palates are at higher risk for hearing issues.

By working closely with a multidisciplinary team of specialists, maintaining good oral hygiene practices, and attending regular checkups, parents can help ensure their child achieves the best possible outcomes in oral health and overall well-being.

The timing of orthodontic treatment for children with cleft lip and palate is determined on a case-by-case basis through consultation. Therefore, it is not possible to specify a standard age at which treatment should begin.

Currently, orthodontic treatment for conditions caused by cleft lip and palate is covered by health insurance, and the number of institutions designated as specialized developmental medical facilities is increasing. Orthodontic treatment is a long-term process. Before starting treatment, it is important to consult with your doctor about the convenience of regular clinic visits, whether the institution is designated as a developmental medical facility, and whether the treatment will be covered by insurance.

Collaborating with kindergarten and elementary school teachers

Surprisingly, many parents do not inform kindergarten or elementary school teachers about their child's medical condition.

As a result, in school settings, children with cleft lip and palate may face challenges such as being scolded by teachers for eating lunch slowly or for unclear speech during reading activities. Some children may not share these experiences with their parents, leading to unnoticed emotional distress. Over time, this can cause the child to develop a dislike for attending kindergarten or school.

To prevent such situations, it is essential to inform teachers about your child's condition, especially during transitions like class changes or promotions. Responding to requests from many parents, the NPO Japan Cleft Lip and Palate Association has created a pamphlet to assist parents in explaining the condition to kindergarten and elementary school teachers. This resource can help foster understanding and support within the school environment.

[Q] 40. WHAT KIND OF TREATMENTS ARE AVAILABLE FOR HIGH SCHOOL AND COLLEGE STUDENTS?

[A] Lip corrective surgery or nasal alar surgery may be performed.

For high school and university students with cleft lip and palate, there are several treatment options available: As they grow older, students may undergo surgery to correct the lip and nose. This is often done after their growth is completed, typically during adolescence or young adulthood. However, even after surgery, there can be some changes to the nose's appearance as it continues to develop. After correcting the lip, some of adolescence may still have nasal deformities. These are typically addressed once their facial bones have fully developed to avoid issues like asymmetry or flattening of the nose over time. It's common for scarring and misalignment of the lip border to occur after surgery.

In some cases, if there is not enough tissue in the upper lip, tissue may be transplanted from the lower lip or other areas of the body. Sometimes, artificial appliances or tissues are used to help with the correction.

Maxilla and facial deformities

If the upper jaw (maxilla) has not developed properly or there are occlusion issues from earlier surgeries, treatment will be performed after the jaw growth is complete. This may include jaw surgery and orthodontic treatment. Your dentist will provide a thorough explanation of each treatment option's advantages and disadvantages.

Orthodontic and prosthodontic treatments

Orthodontic care can help expand the alveolar arch (the area of the upper jaw that holds the teeth). In some cases, bone grafts may be performed in the cleft area to support the placement of dental implants. This is typically done by specialists in dental university hospitals or affiliated hospitals. If teeth or parts of the jaw are missing, prosthetic treatments such as dentures, artificial jaws, or implants may be used to restore function and appearance. Unfortunately, some prosthetic treatments may not be covered by health insurance, but efforts are being made to have these treatments included in insurance coverage.

55

CHAPTER 2. PRE-SURGERY AND SURGERY

[Q] 41. IS IT POSSIBLE TO PERFORM BONE GRAFTING OR DISTRACTION OSTEOGENESIS SIMULTANEOUSLY WITH REVISION SURGERY?

[A] **To our knowledge, there are few facilities that perform above surgeries at the same time.**

For children with cleft lip and palate, multiple surgeries are often needed over the years as they grow. Parents and guardians usually want to minimize the number of surgeries, and there are treatments that focus on both the bone structure and soft tissues. There is no set rule for when to perform lip and nose revision surgeries. However, they are generally done before the child enters elementary school or after growth has completed. The goal is to improve the appearance and function of the lips and nose once the body has finished growing.

Some surgeries focus on correcting the bones of the upper jaw (maxilla) and face. For example, bone grafting: This is done to the alveolar area (the part of the jaw where the teeth sit) when the permanent teeth start to come in.

Upper Jaw Correction Surgery (including distraction osteogenesis): This is performed for developmental issues with the maxilla (upper jaw) once the child's growth has finished, typically during adolescence. At a younger age, the bones of the face haven't fully developed, so it's not the best time to address bone issues. Soft tissue corrections like lip or nose shaping may be performed, but bone-related surgeries are usually delayed until after growth is complete. When the child's facial skeletal bone is fully developed, it's the right time for more significant surgeries like bone grafting or osteotomy (cutting and reshaping bones). However, because the shape of the lips and nose depends on the skeletal bone's underneath, these changes can be difficult to predict and plan for at the same time. This is why it is rare for both bone surgeries and soft tissue revision surgeries to be done together. Regarding nasal deformities, in some cases, cartilage from areas like the ribs, hip bones, or ear may be used to fix nasal deformities. This helps support the nose and improve its shape.

[Q] 42. PROVIDE INFORMATION ON THE ADVANTAGES AND DISADVANTAGES OF PHARYNGEAL FLAP SURGERY, INCLUDING THE PROCEDURE, RECOVERY TIME, AND POTENTIAL RISKS

[A] **Pharyngeal flap surgery is a procedure used to improve speech in children who have had cleft palate surgery but the decision as to whether to undergo surgery must be made carefully since it changes the original shape of the pharynx.**

It provides the most stable results for those with a condition called velopharyngeal insufficiency, which causes speech to sound nasal because the soft palate (the back part of the roof of the mouth) does not fully close off the nasal passage when speaking. This is often due to the muscles of the soft palate not moving properly, or the throat being deeper than usual, preventing the soft palate from reaching the back wall of the throat. If speech therapy and other methods do not correct the problem, surgery may be needed.

If a child around age 4 still struggles with speech or has issues like air leaking through the nose when saying certain sounds, tests like a cephalogram or nasopharyngeal endoscopy will be done to check the soft palate and the shape of the throat. During the surgery, a small part of the tissue from the back wall of the throat is attached to the soft palate. This makes it easier for the soft palate to move up and touch the back of the throat when speaking, reducing the nasal sound in speech. While this procedure is effective, it does change the shape of the throat, and it's important to consider the possible side effects.

Possible side effects of pharyngeal flap surgery: Some children report a sense of nasal congestion or discomfort after the surgery, which may make it harder to insert a breathing tube during anesthesia. Also, the back of the throat becomes narrower, which could increase snoring or rarely cause breathing problems, like sleep apnea (when breathing temporarily stops during sleep).

There is also a small risk that it could lead to ear infections, as nasal mucus may not flow down the throat as easily. These issues usually improve within a month, and regular checkups with an ear, nose, and throat doctor (otolaryngologist) can help manage and reduce the risks of ear infections.

CHAPTER 2. PRE-SURGERY AND SURGERY

Q 43. ALVEOLAR BONE GRAFTING, ADVANTAGES AND LIMITATIONS AND THE TIMING OF THE PROCEDURE

A **It is generally performed around the age of 8-12. The advantages and disadvantages are summarized below.**

What is cleft alveolar bone and related problems?

Cleft alveolar bone grafting is a surgical procedure performed to help close gaps in the upper jaw (the alveolar ridge) in children born with a cleft lip and palate. This procedure is typically done when the child is between 8 and 12 years old, but in some cases, it may be done earlier.

About the advantages, disadvantages

Cleft alveolar bone grafting involves filling in the gap (cleft) in the upper jaw with bone, which is usually taken from the iliac bone (a bone from the pelvis). This surgery helps in creating a solid base for teeth to emerge, especially the canine (cuspid) or lateral incisor teeth, which may have difficulty erupting in children with cleft conditions. It also improves the alignment of the teeth with orthodontic treatment.

Advantages of cleft alveolar bone grafting:
   -The bone graft can help improve the shape of the base of the nose.
   -It helps in forming the continuous alveolar ridge (the area where the teeth sit), which stabilizes the upper jaw and ensures the proper eruption of teeth.
   -With the bone in place, teeth can be moved more effectively through orthodontic treatment, especially the canine and lateral incisor teeth.
   - Helps create a proper space for teeth to emerge and grow in the right direction.
Disadvantages and challenges:
   -If there is not enough space for the graft, the procedure may not be as effective. Additionally, if there is a fistula (an opening between the mouth and nose), food and liquids may leak into the nose, and air may leak when speaking.

Timing

Bone grafting is often done when the child reaches the age of 8-12 years, after the growth of the upper jaw is mostly complete. However, some centers may perform this procedure earlier, depending on the individual's needs.

Bone grafting

The bone used for the graft typically comes from the iliac bone (from the pelvis). This means

58

there is a second surgery to collect the bone, which can be uncomfortable and requires recovery time. Incomplete closure: In some cases, the mouth and nasal cavity may not be completely closed after the graft, requiring additional treatments.

When is cleft alveolar bone grafting performed?

Bone grafting is often done in late adolescence or early adulthood when the facial bones are more fully developed. Some facilities may offer earlier bone grafting, but the timing is generally determined based on the growth stage and the individual needs of the patient.

Q 44. WHAT IS ALVEOLAR CLEFT BONE GRAFTING?

A This procedure is undertaken to enhance the alignment of the teeth.

Alveolar bone grafting is a surgical procedure aimed at improving the alignment of teeth in children with cleft lip and palate. It helps close gaps in the upper jaw (maxilla) where teeth are missing or misaligned, providing a better foundation for future tooth development and orthodontic treatment.

The surgery often involves using bone from the child's own body, typically the iliac bone (a bone from the lower back), as it is a good source for transplantation. However, other materials, such as artificial materials or bone from another person, may also be used depending on the child's needs. This procedure is usually performed between the ages of 7 and 12, when the teeth are emerging and the jaw is still developing.

It is often done in conjunction with orthodontic treatment to help move the teeth into proper alignment after the bone graft is placed. Since alveolar bone grafting is related to other surgeries, the timing and materials used can vary, making it important for parents to consult with their doctor to determine the best course of action for their child. For additional support and guidance, organizations like the Japanese Cleft Lip and Palate Foundation offer consultations to help address any concerns. Reception hours: Monday to Friday: 10:00-16:00. TEL:052-757-4312

CHAPTER 2. PRE-SURGERY AND SURGERY

Q 45. IS IT POSSIBLE TO PUT IMPLANTS IN REPLACEMENT BONES? PLEASE EXPLAIN THE ACTUAL METHOD?

A **Recently, alveolar bone grafting has been incorporated into comprehensive treatment, making it possible to use implants for missing lateral incisors.**

Yes, implants can be placed on bone that has been grafted, and this is becoming a common part of the treatment for children with cleft lip and palate. After the bone grafting procedure, implants can be used to replace missing teeth, particularly for the lateral incisor, which is the second tooth from the front.

However, this process involves several steps and requires careful planning. Initially, after bone grafting, orthodontic treatment is often performed to align the teeth and create the proper space for the implant. In some cases, a healthy adjacent tooth may need to be slightly shaved to make room for the implant. The implant procedure itself is usually done under local anesthesia and does not require hospitalization.

ACT scan is often done to check the condition of the bone, ensuring there is enough height and width in the jaw to support the implant. Once the bone graft has had time to heal and the proper conditions are met, an implant fixture (which acts as the root of the tooth) can be placed in the bone. The gums are carefully incised to expose the grafted bone, and the implant is inserted into the bone. This process typically takes about a year, as the bone needs time to integrate with the implant. Afterward, a crown is mounted on the implant.

For patients with cleft lip and palate, bone grafting is often performed first, followed by the implant placement after several months or even years, as the graft needs time to fully take hold. Some patients may require additional bone grafting or procedures to restore the shape and function of the teeth and upper jaw.

Although implants are a more permanent solution for missing teeth, they are not always covered by insurance, and their cost can be high. Insurance coverage for implant procedures varies depending on the facility and specific treatment plans. Recently, there has been movement to make implants more accessible for cleft lip and palate patients, and some university hospitals and approved dental institutions may offer implant treatments as part of advanced medical care.

In summary, implants can be placed on grafted bone, but the process is complex and requires careful planning, including bone grafting, orthodontic treatment, and several surgical steps. Parents should consult with their dental team to determine the best approach based on their child's specific needs and condition.

60

Q 46. IS IT POSSIBLE TO HAVE BONE GRAFTING FOR ADULTS?

A **Bone grafting is typically done around the age of 8, just before the maxillary lateral incisors (the teeth next to the front teeth) or age 10 when maxillary canines (the pointed teeth next to the lateral incisors) are about to come in.**

While bone grafting can technically be done at any time, it is most effective when performed before these teeth emerge. The reason for this is that the bone in the area of a cleft may not be strong enough to support these teeth as they come in, and the bone may become absorbed or weakened over time. If the bone is not strong enough for implants, bone grafting can still be done later, even after a person has reached adulthood. However, it's generally better to perform the graft before the teeth grow in to ensure the best results. In some cases, if the alveolar bone is not sufficient for implant placement, a bone graft can be performed even after reaching adulthood, but the earlier this is done, the more successful the treatment is likely to be. The goal is to help stabilize the teeth and ensure they are properly aligned with the alveolar bone of the jaw. Typically, this procedure is carried out at the age of 8, before the second maxillary incisors erupts, or at the age of 10, coinciding with the eruption of the canines, as highlighted earlier.

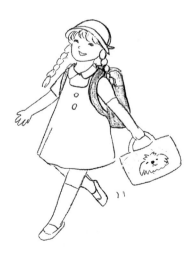

CHAPTER 2. PRE-SURGERY AND SURGERY

[Q] 47. PLEASE SHARE ABOUT REGENERATIVE TREATMENT AND ITS ADVANTAGES DURING ALVEOLAR BONE TRANSPLANTATION

[A] **Regenerative medicine refers to medical treatment that uses cultured tissue or stem cells to repair missing or damaged organs and tissues. If clinical application of IPS cells advances in the future, skin, mucous membranes, and dental pulp may also be used as donors.**

This process has been used for skin, corneas, cartilage, and other tissues. Stem cells are special cells that can develop into many different types of cells in the body. There are different types of stem cells, including embryonic stem cells (ES cells) and induced pluripotent stem cells (iPS cells), which are created by altering adult cells (like skin or mucous membrane cells) to become pluripotent—meaning they can turn into various kinds of tissues or organs. However, iPS cells and ES cells are still in the early stages of research, and are not yet widely used in medical practice because it's difficult to obtain them and the technology is still being developed. On the other hand, tissue stem cells are specialized to form certain types of cells, such as blood cells or nerve cells. One example of this is hematopoietic stem cells, which are used to treat blood-related cancers like leukemia.

Another application is in bone marrow transplants, where stem cells from the bone marrow are used to treat bone issues, such as those caused by alveolar clefts. Currently, clinical research is looking into how bone marrow stromal cells—which are found in bone marrow—can be cultured and turned into bone-forming cells (osteoblasts). This method shows promise for treating the bone loss or atrophy that occurs in areas like the alveolar ridge in cleft patients. As the use of iPS cells advances, other sources, such as skin, mucous membranes, and dental pulp (from teeth), might also be used as sources of stem cells for regenerative treatments. This research is still in its early stages, but it holds a lot of potential for the future of cleft treatment and many other medical applications.

62

Q 48. CAN YOU TELL ME ABOUT THE TIME AND SURGICAL METHOD OF CLOSING PALATAL FISTULA?

A Palatal fistula closure is a surgical procedure used to close holes in the palate (roof of the mouth) that may remain after cleft palate surgery. This procedure is typically performed when a child reaches the age of 8 to 11, often at the same time as a cleft bone graft.

The timing can vary depending on the specific medical facility, but it is generally done during this age range. The surgery to close a palatal fistula can be done in one session or in two stages. In some cases, the surgery is performed all at once, targeting areas such as the septum (the dividing wall of the nose) or the front of the hard palate. In other cases, the surgery is performed in two stages: the first focuses on the parts of the palate that are essential for speech, and the second stage addresses the front part of the palate to allow for upper jaw development.

For children with a larger cleft, if the fistula is too large to be closed with the palate tissue alone, a tongue flap may be used. This involves taking a small piece of tissue from the tongue to help close the hole in the palate. Although effective, this method can cause additional stress after surgery, as the tongue tissue and palate must be separated after about a week to allow for healing. If a tongue flap is needed, the fistula closure is typically performed starting at around age 15. In some cases, the surgery is combined with bone grafting for the alveolar cleft (the gap in the upper jaw), providing a more comprehensive solution.

While the timing of the surgery can vary depending on the child's specific condition, it generally takes several weeks for the blood supply to the palate and tongue tissue to stabilize, allowing for proper healing. The goal of this surgery is to ensure the best possible function and appearance of the palate, while also supporting speech and upper jaw development.

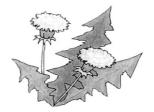

Q 49. WOULD IT BE AVAILABLE FOR ADULTS, WHO HAS CROSSBITE TO BE TREATED?

A **Yes, adult crossbite can be treated, and there are two main types of treatment depending on the cause of the crossbite.**

If the main cause is related to the facial bone structure, surgery is often needed to move the lower jaw (the mandible) back into the correct position to fix the bite.

However, if the problem is not related to the bone structure, treatment typically begins with orthodontics, such as braces or aligners, to realign the teeth. Afterward, if necessary, surgery may be performed to complete the correction.

In both cases, surgery is only applied after a thorough examination by a dentist in the oral and maxillofacial department to ensure the best treatment plan. The dentist will determine whether surgery is required immediately or if orthodontics should be done first.

In summary, adult crossbite can be treated with a combination of orthodontics and surgery, based on the underlying cause, with a dentist guiding the treatment approach after a careful assessment.

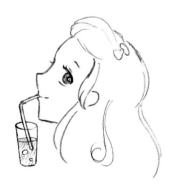

Q 50. WHAT IS CORRECTIVE SURGERY? WHAT TYPES OF SURGERIES ARE EXIST?

A The procedure involves correcting bone structure and occlusion through surgery. These include Le Fort osteotomy, distraction osteogenesis, sagittal split ramus osteotomy, and vertical mandibular osteotomy.

Surgical orthodontic surgery is a procedure used to correct the bone structure and bite. It is often needed for children with cleft lip and palate, especially when the bones of the jaw are not properly aligned. There are different types of surgical orthodontic treatments, each designed for specific bone issues, including type I osteotomy, bone distraction, sagittal split ramus osteotomy (SSRO), and vertical mandibular osteotomy (IVRO). In the case of type I osteotomy, the jawbone is cut and repositioned to correct the bite. Bone distraction involves slowly lengthening the bone over time.

SSRO is used when the lower jaw is too far forward (mandibular prognathism), while IVRO is used when there are issues with the lower jaw's alignment, such as it being too far back or too far forward. These surgeries are often performed when there are problems with the bone structure, like a protruding upper jaw or a protruding lower jaw, which can occur in children with cleft lip and palate. This can be caused by scarring from previous surgeries, which affects how the jaw and face grow. In some cases, a bone lengthening device is used to gradually lengthen the bones in the jaw to correct these issues.

For maxillary retrognathism (when the upper jaw is too far back), bone lengthening devices may be used. There are two types of devices: external and intraoral. External devices are more flexible but can be uncomfortable and harder to use daily, as they require attachment to the head. Intraoral devices are more comfortable but can only lengthen the bone in one direction. Both devices have their limitations, but they help in adjusting the jaw's position.

For mandibular prognathism (when the lower jaw is too far forward), SSRO and IVRO are commonly used. SSRO has the advantage of a shorter recovery time, as the jaw is repositioned using plates and screws, while IVRO does not use screws or plates, making recovery a bit easier, though the bite may take longer to stabilize. Overall, surgical orthodontic treatments for cleft lip and palate patients are customized to each individual's needs. In many cases, a combination of different surgeries is used to achieve the best outcome. While there may be some restrictions on daily life during recovery, these surgeries can greatly improve the bite and overall appearance of the jaw and face.

CHAPTER 2. PRE-SURGERY AND SURGERY

[Q] 51. TELL US ABOUT WHAT IS BONE LENGTHENING SURGERY, ITS INSTRUMENTS AND METHODS AND TIME?

[A] Please read details below.

Bone lengthening is a medical procedure used to gradually increase the length of bones. It involves making a controlled break in a bone (called osteotomy) under anesthesia, and then slowly pulling apart the broken parts to stimulate the growth of new bone in the gap during the healing process.

This new bone growth happens naturally, and over time, the bone becomes longer. This method was first used in orthopedic surgery for limb-lengthening but is now also used in maxillofacial surgery (surgery on the jaw and face) for conditions like cleft lip and palate. Bone lengthening involves using a special device to slowly extend the bone. There are two types of devices: external devices and intraoral devices. External devices are attached outside the body and are visible, often requiring pins to be placed in the head for support. These devices offer more flexibility in bone lengthening but can be uncomfortable and cause some limitations in daily life.

Intraoral devices are smaller and are placed inside the mouth, under the gum, with only a rotating screw visible. These devices are less noticeable and cause fewer restrictions, but surgery is needed to remove the device after the lengthening process is complete. The amount and direction of bone lengthening that can be achieved with the intraoral device are more limited compared to external devices.

The bone lengthening process typically starts with surgery to cut the bone and attach the device. After the surgery, the device is used to gradually lengthen the bone. The extension usually begins about a week after the surgery, with the bone being lengthened at a rate of about 0.5 to 1 millimeter per day. Once the planned lengthening is achieved, the device stays in place until the new bone has fully formed and healed, which can take several (around 3) months.

While this procedure is generally safe and effective for treating jaw growth issues in cleft lip and palate patients, it is important to follow the doctor's advice to ensure the best results and avoid complications. Overall, bone lengthening is a reliable treatment option for certain jaw development issues related to cleft lip and palate. If your doctor recommends it, you can feel confident in considering it as a safe and effective treatment.

Q 52. IS IT POSSIBLE TO MAKE SCARS FROM CLEFT LIP SURGERY LESS NOTICEABLE?

A Yes, it is possible to make scars from cleft lip surgery less noticeable, although they may not disappear completely. One way to reduce the appearance of scars is by using cosmetics, particularly foundation as a base makeup. Products like Covermark, which are commercially available, are designed to help cover scars by suppressing redness and smoothing out unevenness in the skin.

However, it's important to note that scars may still be visible depending on the lighting and skin type. After surgery, doctors can provide counseling to help prevent the formation of hypertrophic scars, which are raised, reddish, and more noticeable than regular scars.

These types of scars can be painful and itchy. In some cases, even if a scar is surgically removed, new scars can form, especially if someone is prone to hypertrophic scars (also known as keloids).

To treat these, oral medications like tranilast (an anti-allergy drug) or topical steroids can be used over time to reduce their appearance, but they may still remain visible. To help with this, using cosmetics such as foundation can also improve the appearance of the skin, making scars look more natural. This can help reduce mental discomfort by making the scars less noticeable.

There are products, such as sebum (a cosmetic developed in the United States), that can be used to naturally hide scars and bruises, providing additional coverage.

References
1) GRAFA Laboratories http://www.grafa.jp/individual/
2) COVERMARK http://www.covermark.co.jp/shop/

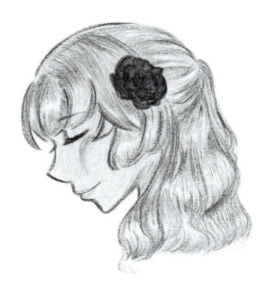

67

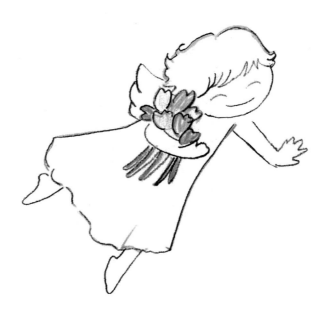

CHAPTER 3. ORTHODONTICS, PROSTHODONTICS

Q 53. IS PATIENTS WITH CLEFTS SUSPECTED TO HAVE CROSSBITE?

A No, it doesn't mean that every child with clefts to have crossbite.

Children with cleft lip and palate are not necessarily more likely to develop mandibular prognathism or crossbite (a condition where the lower jaw protrudes forward). However, in some cases, the lower jaw may appear more forward than usual due to the periosteum (a layer of tissue) of the hard palate. This can happen if the upper jaw does not grow properly, even after treatment. The development of the lower jaw may be influenced by factors such as scarring from surgery, increased pressure on the lips due to the cleft lip closure, and developmental issues in the upper jaw. These factors can cause the upper jaw to not grow as expected, which can lead to maxillary retrognathism.

Children with cleft lip and palate are regularly monitored by pediatric dentists and oral surgeons, starting at an early age. X-rays and regular checkups allow the doctors to track how the jaw is developing. If necessary, orthodontic treatment is performed at the right time to help with jaw alignment, and techniques like maxillary forward traction can be used to help the upper jaw grow properly. In most cases, by the time the child reaches adulthood, the occlusion (bite) improves.

However, if the occlusion doesn't improve on its own as the child grows, surgery (called osteotomy) may be performed on both the upper and lower jaws after the growth stops to correct the bite.

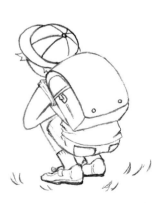

[Q] 54. WILL A CHILD WITH CLEFT LIP AND PALATE DEVELOP TEETH MISALIGNMENT, AND IS ORTHODONTIC TREATMENT INEVITABLE?

[A] **Children with cleft lip and palate are more likely to have misaligned teeth. In addition, orthodontic treatment is necessary to support maxillary growth and development.**

Cleft lip and palate are congenital conditions that occur when specific tissues in certain parts of the craniofacial region are absent or underdeveloped. Depending on which part of the face is affected, the condition is classified into two main types.

If only a part of the lip is missing, the condition is referred to as **cleft lip**. When the cleft extends into the upper jaw (the maxilla), it is classified as **cleft lip and alveolus**.

The second type involves a cleft in the **palate**, specifically in the roof of the mouth (palatal region). This condition is termed **cleft palate**. If both the lip and the palate are affected simultaneously, it is called **cleft lip and palate**.

In all these cases, surgical intervention is necessary to close the gap by pulling surrounding tissues together and stitching them to repair the defect. Since tissue from the surrounding areas is used to fill the missing parts, the process of stitching these tissues together can result in the formation of scar tissue. This scarring can inhibit normal growth and development in the affected area, which may impact the alignment of the teeth and facial structure in the future and lead to malocclusion.

In some cases, an opposite overbite may be observed in the molar region. However, surgical intervention may not always be necessary. For certain visible defects in the palate, language therapy alone may be sufficient. In cases of isolated cleft lip or cleft lip with alveolus, surgery results in the loss of the softness of the upper lip, which pushes the upper front teeth backward. However, the impact rarely extends to the molar region, and it is unlikely that the baby molars will exhibit an overbite. Regarding cleft palate, particularly submucosal cleft palate, it is often enough to treat the condition with speech therapy alone. When defects are present, there are currently two main approaches to treatment.

In mild cases of cleft lip, orthodontic treatment may be required. In cases where speech therapy is unnecessary, one treatment approach prioritizes "surgery to acquire language" before the child reaches the age of 6 years. For cases of cleft lip and palate with cleft lip and alveolus, surgery is performed when the child reaches a weight of **6 kg**, followed by palatal surgery when the child reaches a weight of **10 kg**. This is the most common treatment approach.

In such surgeries, early palatal reconstruction can cause scarring, which may interfere with the growth and development of the upper jaw (maxilla). As a result, orthodontic treatment becomes necessary to compensate for the disruption of normal growth. However, in this case, the focus of orthodontic treatment is not on aligning the teeth, but rather on correcting the upper jaw. This in-

71

CHAPTER 3. ORTHODONTICS, PROSTHODONTICS

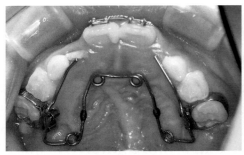

Fig. 1   Lateral expansion appliance

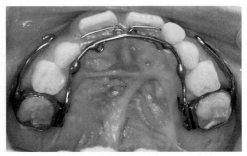

Fig. 2   Attachments for the anterior expansion appliance and protraction appliance

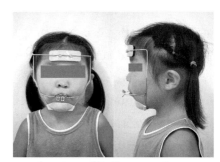

Fig. 3   With the maxillary protraction device in place

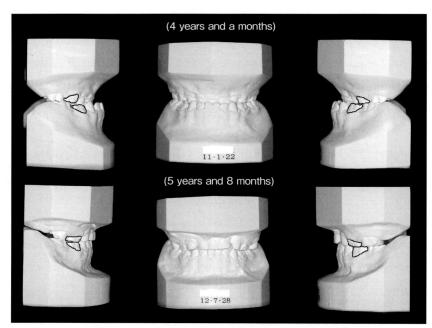

Fig. 4   Before and after using anterior protraction device

Case 1:

The first deciduous molar has shifted forward, resulting in an improvement in the anterior teeth's overjet.

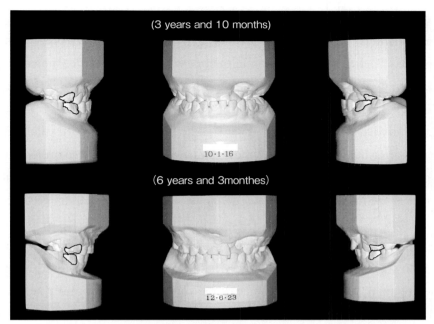

Fig. 5 Before and after using maxillary protraction device

Case 2:
The first deciduous molar has shifted mesially, resulting in improved overbite and coverage of the anterior teeth.

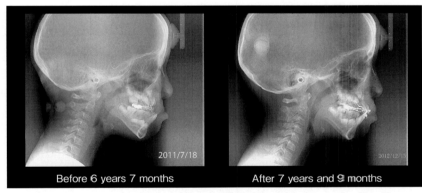

Fig. 6 A comparison of the soft tissue before and after the application of an anterior protraction device shows that the upper lip's concavity has been corrected

volves orthodontic treatment aimed at restoring the normal growth of a delayed upper jaw (maxilla). Specifically, the maxilla, which is being pulled back due to palatal scarring (with both sides of the baby molars showing an opposite overbite), is expanded laterally, and the underdeveloped upper jaw is moved forward. In many cases of cleft lip and alveolus, orthodontic treatment is performed to correct the growth and development of the upper jaw.

When you look at the faces of children with clefts, the upper jaw often appears underdeveloped, and the lower jaw does not protrude. Instead, the upper lip looks sunken, giving the initial impression that the lower jaw is protruding forward. If surgery is performed with a focus on language acquisition, orthodontic treatment of the jaw, starting at the age of 4 or 5, can significantly improve the future development of the midface.

This approach is crucial for addressing maxillary hypoplasia commonly observed in patients with cleft lip and palate. Traditionally, orthodontic treatment was initiated after the eruption of permanent dentition, aligning the teeth but often leaving a concave midfacial profile. Currently, maxillary expansion (**Fig. 1**) is initiated around the age of 4 to 5 years and 2 months, followed by anterior expansion of the maxillary dentition (**Fig. 2**) and stimulation of forward maxillary growth using a protraction headgear or other protrusive traction appliances (**Fig. 3**). These orthodontic treatments, referred to as dentoalveolar and maxillary orthopedic interventions, are designed to guide the growth and development of the maxilla in children with clefts. **Fig. 4 to 6** illustrate the outcomes of these treatment approaches.

Another treatment approach for children with cleft lip and palate involves performing lip closure surgery first, followed by palate closure surgery before the age of 6. However, when palatoplasty is delayed, the "optimal" functional outcomes of the surgery may not be fully achieved. Although maxillary underdevelopment may be less pronounced in such cases, it does not eliminate the need for further correction, as growth potential remains. Additionally, while the goal is to complete speech acquisition by the age of 6, the persistence of a palatal fistula often leads to challenges in achieving optimal speech outcomes.

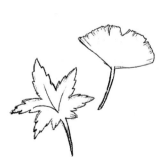

Q 55. I WAS TOLD NOT TO LET MY CHILD GET CAVITIES FOR THE SAKE OF FUTURE ORTHODONTIC TREATMENT. WHY IS THAT?

A This is because inadequate oral hygiene, with cavities makes it unsuitable to apply a multi-bracket appliance. Furthermore, during orthodontic treatment with a multi-bracket appliance, which is associated with an increased risk of dental caries, it is crucial to ensure that the patient is adequately prepared to manage their oral hygiene independently, including proper brushing and other preventive measures, to avoid the development of caries.

Dental caries, or cavities, develop when food debris accumulates on teeth and forms a habitat for cariogenic bacteria in dental plaque. These bacteria, such as *Streptococcus mutans*, multiply and produce acidic substances from sugars, leading to demineralization of enamel and the dissolution of the hard structure of the teeth.

If cavities progress, the dental pulp, commonly referred to as the tooth nerve, may need to be removed. In severe cases, tooth extraction may become necessary. Therefore, regardless of whether orthodontic treatment is undertaken, preventing cavities is critical.

In children with cleft lip and palate, anatomical challenges such as maxillary clefts and surgical interventions can lead to maxillary hypoplasia, particularly in the anterior and lateral regions. This frequently results in a smaller maxilla and severe dental crowding.

To prevent cavities, especially during orthodontic treatment, proper oral hygiene is essential. This includes plaque control, fluoride use, and brushing habits. Establishing habits such as brushing after meals and before bed, as well as reducing the intake of sugary snacks and beverages, is critical.

During the mixed dentition stage, when many teeth are transitioning from primary to permanent dentition, enamel immaturity and inadequate plaque control increase the risk of cavities. Parental assistance with brushing is especially important at this stage.

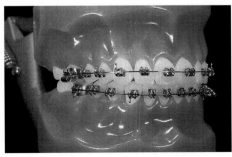

Fig. 1 Multi-bracket appliance (metal)

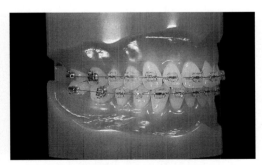

Fig. 2 Multi-bracket appliance (non-metal)

For children with clefts, orthodontic treatment using multi-bracket appliances (**Fig. 1, 2**) can be complex and prolonged. These appliances create an environment where plaque and food debris can accumulate, increasing the risk of cavities. Preventive care, including fluoride application and professional cleaning, is essential during this time to maintain a healthy oral environment.

One key objective of preventing cavities before starting orthodontic treatment is to ensure that the child with clefts is prepared to manage their own oral hygiene, including effective brushing. This preparation reduces the risk of cavities during treatment with multi-bracket appliances. If a child has multiple cavities in their permanent teeth or poor oral hygiene due to untreated cavities before starting orthodontic treatment, the placement of multi-bracket appliances may not be possible. Such situations can lead to treatment delays or interruptions, and in severe cases, orthodontic treatment may need to be canceled entirely.

Maintaining good oral hygiene before treatment not only helps preserve as many healthy teeth as possible for the future but also ensures that orthodontic treatment proceeds smoothly. For these reasons, both the child and their caregivers must prioritize oral hygiene. Caregivers, in particular, play a crucial role by assisting with tasks such as final brushing until the patient has mastered proper brushing techniques. Careful attention to oral hygiene and cavity prevention is essential.

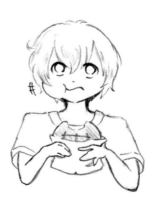

[Q] 56. PLEASE PROVIDE INFORMATION ABOUT THE COST OF ORTHODONTIC TREATMENT AND AVAILABLE PUBLIC SUBSIDIES

[A] **The cost of orthodontic treatment can be high, especially for children with cleft lip and palate. Therefore, it is important to make use of the available support systems. Depending on the household income and the municipality of residence, the types and extent of public subsidies available may vary. To get detailed information, please contact the relevant department in your local municipality.**

The cost of general orthodontic treatment, will be considered "optional medical treatment" (self-paid treatment) and will not be covered by insurance. However, if you have a medical condition designated by the Ministry of Health, Labor and Welfare of Japan (47 diseases), including cleft lip and palate, orthodontic treatment for occlusion abnormalities caused by dental issues (as of April 2014), and treatment for jaw deformities requiring surgery, including pre- and post-operative orthodontic care, are covered by health insurance. The patient is responsible for 30% of the medical expenses as a self-payment.

Additionally, patients requiring orthodontic treatment to improve speech, voice, language, and chewing function disorders caused by cleft lip and palate are eligible for public assistance through the Independent Medical Support System, which reduces the self-payment amount for medical expenses.

The system unifies the procedures and payment mechanisms of the three public medical care systems for disabilities—namely "developmental medical care," "rehabilitation medical care," and "mental outpatient medical care"—which were previously separate systems under the Act. It became one unified system in April 2006. If an application is made and medical support is approved, the patient's out-of-pocket expenses will be reduced by a certain percentage. Additionally, further reduction measures are implemented to prevent out-of-pocket expenses from becoming excessive, and a maximum monthly out-of-pocket amount is set based on income.

When a patient with clefts is eligible for the medical assistance system, they must apply for either "Medical Assistance for Independence (Developmental Medical Assistance)" or "Medical Assistance for Independence (Rehabilitation Medical Assistance)" depending on the child's age. "Developmental Medical Assistance" is intended for children under the age of 18 with physical disabilities who can benefit from treatments such as surgery to remove or reduce their disabilities. "Rehabilitation Medical Assistance" is available to individuals aged 18 or older with physical disabilities. However, it is important to note that when applying, the individual must have a disability certificate issued in accordance with the Welfare of Persons with Disabilities Act. Additionally, in order to receive assistance with medical expenses for these independent living support services, the medical institution must be designated as a developmental or rehabilitation medical institution.

The documents required for the application are available at your local health center or city hall. Please fill out the necessary information and submit your application. Even after approval, you will need to continue submitting applications every six months to a year. Treatment for cleft lip and palate requires the cooperation of specialists from various fields, such as oral surgery, plastic surgery, prosthetics, and orthodontics, to provide consistent care. As the treatment is long-term, the cost can be high. Therefore, we recommend utilizing these systems; however, please note that there are limitations to the Support Medical Care based on the family's annual income. If your income exceeds the limit, the self-payment rate will be 10%, and you will only need to pay this percentage each month.

The maximum copayment amount does not apply. Additionally, your local municipality may provide public medical assistance for children, in addition to the assistance available for persons with disabilities. For example, if your municipality does not charge medical expenses for children up to junior high school age, you may not need to apply for medical assistance for persons with disabilities until eligibility is reached. In any case, the type of public assistance available and the amount of assistance you can receive will vary depending on your household income and the municipality you live in. For further details, please contact the relevant department in your city or town.

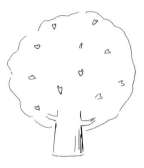

Q 57. WHEN IS THE OPTIMAL TIME TO BEGIN ORTHODONTIC TREATMENT FOR CHILDREN WITH CLEFT LIP AND PALATE, AND HOW LONG WILL IT TAKE?

A Orthodontic treatment for children with cleft lip and palate is a long-term process, and it is important not to start it too early. However, there are optimal periods for starting treatment to correct jaw misalignment and perform alveolar bone grafts (surgery to close gaps in the jaw), so it's crucial to begin treatment when the timing is right based on the child's development and the condition of their malocclusion (bite problems). It's best to consult an orthodontist to determine the best time for starting treatment and to get an overview of the process.

For children with cleft lip and palate, the upper jaw may not develop properly due to the effects of surgery, leading to underdevelopment of the upper jaw, which can cause crooked or crowded teeth. In these cases, orthodontic treatment is typically started around age 5, but it depends on the child's growth and the condition of their teeth.

Another important consideration in orthodontic treatment for cleft lip and palate is the presence of a cleft in the alveolar ridge. This cleft creates a communication between the mouth and the nasal cavity, which can result in nasal leakage of food or fluids, and may lead to relapses in orthodontic alignment after treatment. Additionally, the lateral incisors and canines may fail to erupt in the correct position due to insufficient bone structure in the affected area.

This can cause damage to the maxilla. Furthermore, if there is bone loss, it is impossible to move the teeth into that area, and ultimately gaps will remain between the teeth. For this reason, bone grafts, such as from the iliac crest, have been performed in recent years into the alveolar cleft area. Closing the alveolar cleft makes it possible to move the teeth into that area, allowing the patient to achieve tooth alignment without gaps using their own teeth. It is believed that relapse after maxillary expansion is unlikely to occur. Although there are individual differences in bone grafting, when it is performed around the age of 8 to 10, when the canine teeth begin to erupt, the grafted bone usually integrates well. The overall condition is also considered favorable. Therefore, it is essential to complete maxillary expansion before performing alveolar bone grafting, as the timing of the grafting is closely related to the initiation of orthodontic treatment. After the first phase of treatment is completed, a second evaluation is typically conducted around 12-13 years of age to assess the extent of improvement in jaw alignment.

Additionally, since many cases involve morphological abnormalities and congenitally missing teeth, the final treatment plan, including orthodontic management, is not determined at this stage. This includes deciding how the permanent dentition should be aligned. For instance, after encouraging forward growth of the maxilla using a maxillary protraction device, it is evaluated whether the skeletal mandibular prognathism has improved and whether sufficient space for proper tooth alignment has been created by lateral expansion of the maxilla with an expansion device.

If the first phase of treatment is successfully completed, the second phase of treatment can often be achieved using orthodontic methods alone, without the need for tooth extractions. However, in cases where significant mandibular overgrowth occurs or the discrepancy between tooth size and jaw size remains unresolved, additional interventions may be required. This could include surgical orthodontic treatment involving jaw osteotomy or the extraction of permanent teeth to ensure proper alignment and harmony between the dentition and jaw size.

The second stage of orthodontic treatment typically begins after the age of 12-13, once all permanent teeth have erupted. This stage involves the gradual application of a "multi-bracket appliance" to the teeth. Given the complexity of this phase, a minimum treatment period of 2-3 years is required, meaning orthodontic treatment may be completed around the age of 15-16 at the earliest.

In boys, the mandible experiences a growth spurt approximately 2-3 years later than in girls. Therefore, in cases of skeletal mandibular prognathism, terminating treatment before the completion of growth may result in recurrence of mandibular prognathism. For this reason, treatment for boys may need to continue until around the age of 18, when growth is nearly complete.

Once tooth alignment is achieved, the multi-bracket appliance is removed, but retention is necessary to maintain the achieved results. A thin wire retainer is typically bonded to the lingual (inner) surface of the teeth, or a removable retainer is provided. Regular follow-ups are crucial during this retention phase. Retainer treatment is usually required for approximately two years to prevent relapse and maintain the alignment of the teeth (**Fig. 1**).

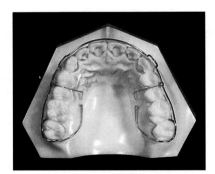

Fig. 1   Retention device

Orthodontic treatment does not end quickly, even if started early. The ultimate goal is to align the permanent dentition and establish an optimal occlusion, which can sometimes require more than 10 years. Variations in treatment duration can occur depending on the type and severity of the cleft, such as whether the patient has a cleft lip, cleft palate, or both. Factors such as the cleft's location, the extent of the alveolar cleft, and whether the patient has other dental anomalies (e.g., congenitally missing teeth) can significantly influence treatment planning and duration. Additionally, genetic predispositions inherited from parents may contribute to variations in tooth alignment, further impacting the timing and specifics of orthodontic intervention.

While orthodontic treatment for cleft lip and palate patients requires a long-term commitment, starting treatment unnecessarily early is not advised. Instead, it is crucial to identify optimal periods for addressing jaw misalignment and performing alveolar bone grafting to ensure effective outcomes. Missing these critical periods could compromise the results of treatment.

At orthodontic consultations, we provide thorough evaluations of occlusion and alignment, as well as counseling tailored to the patient's specific condition. The timing of treatment initiation and an individualized treatment outline will be determined based on the patient's malocclusion and growth patterns. For further information and a detailed procedural plan, please consult with your orthodontist.

Q 58. SHOULD TEETH WITH ABNORMAL MORPHOLOGY OR MALPOSITION THAT HAVE ERUPTED IN THE CLEFT AREA BE EXTRACTED EARLY?

A **It is important to avoid extracting teeth prematurely without careful consideration. However, if the position of the teeth is problematic and interferes with alveolar bone grafting surgery, or if they create an unclean area that could lead to postoperative infections, extraction may be necessary.**

It is generally recommended to avoid extracting teeth too easily, even if they are abnormally shaped or in an incorrect position. However, if a tooth is positioned poorly and it interferes with necessary treatments, like bone grafting, or if it creates an area that could lead to infection after surgery, it may be necessary to extract the tooth. In the area of the arytenoid (a part of the mouth affected by clefts), the lateral incisors (the fourth teeth from the front) often have an unusual shape, such as being cone-shaped or plug-shaped, and they tend to be smaller than normal. In some cases, these teeth may be missing from birth. Additionally, because of bone loss in the arytenoid area, these teeth (including canines) may not grow in the proper position and may shift to the back of the mouth, a condition called lingual displacement. In the past, when bone grafting wasn't as commonly used, malformed teeth were often extracted because the lack of bone support in the arytenoid area prevented the teeth from being moved into their correct positions.

However, even in cases of malformed teeth, their roots are often similar to those of healthy teeth. If these teeth are treated with dental implants or covered with appropriate materials, they can function just like normal teeth. With bone grafting, it is possible to reposition the teeth and guide them into their correct position in the jaw. In fact, keeping the lateral incisors can help improve the success rate of bone grafting.

While it's possible to extract teeth at any time, it's important to note that once a tooth is removed, it can't be replaced. Therefore, even for teeth with abnormal positioning or shape, it's best to avoid

81

CHAPTER 3. ORTHODONTICS, PROSTHODONTICS

extraction unless necessary. If a tooth is causing problems with the bone grafting procedure or is in a position that makes it hard to keep the area clean, which could lead to infection after surgery, extraction might be required. In orthodontic treatment, sometimes premolars (the smaller molars) are removed to create space for the teeth to align properly.

However, when considering extractions, especially for teeth with shape or position issues, it's important to think about the long-term outcome, such as how the permanent teeth will fit together, and to discuss it with the orthodontist. If teeth remain in the cleft area, they are more likely to get stained or develop cavities, so maintaining oral hygiene is very important. In any case, teeth in the cleft area should be carefully examined by an orthodontist before making a final decision about extraction or treatment. A detailed treatment plan should be developed to ensure the best outcome for your child's oral health and development.

Q 59. DOES ORTHODONTIC TREATMENT CREATE OR ENLARGE A HOLE IN THE PALATE?

A In some cases, a hole in the palate may be noticeable. However, by attaching an obturator to the expansion device, there are no issues in daily life.

Orthodontic treatment generally does not cause new holes in the palate, but in some cases, a small hole that was not noticed before may become more visible or slightly larger during the process of lateral expansion (widening of the jaw). This is due to the movement of the teeth and jaw, which can cause an existing hole, known as a fistula, to become more noticeable. However, to prevent this from affecting daily life, a closure plate can be attached to the expansion device during treatment (**Fig.1**).

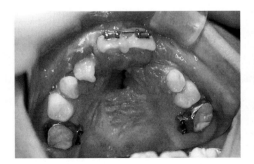 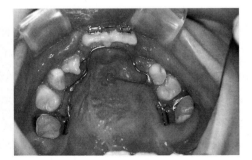

Fig. 1 Attaching the closure plate to the orthodontic appliance and closing the hole

This plate helps close the hole and ensures that there are no significant changes to your child's daily routine or comfort. In cases where there is a hole in the palate, fistula closure surgery is typically done along with bone grafting during the orthodontic treatment. This procedure helps close the hole permanently while ensuring that the treatment progresses smoothly without any complications.

[Q] 60. PLEASE TELL ME ABOUT IMPLANTS FOR CLEFT LIP AND PALATE

[Q] How much does it cost?

[A] **The general cost for a single tooth implant is approximately 300,000 to 400,000 yen. For patients with cleft lip and palate, the cost may be around 300,000 yen.**

Dental implants, which are embedded in the jawbone, are primarily classified into two components: the implant body (artificial dental root) and the abutment (artificial dental crown) (**Fig. 1**).

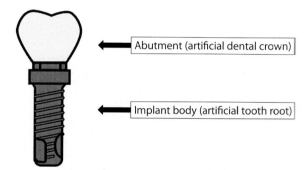

Fig. 1   Components of implant

The implant body is typically constructed from titanium or titanium alloy and may be coated with hydroxyapatite, a biocompatible material with a composition analogous to that of bone. There are several hundred implant manufacturers globally.

The price of dental implants varies depending on the manufacturer and country of origin. The abutment is then connected to the implant body using various connection methods, and there are several types of abutments available, such as metal bond (ceramic fused to a metal crown), all-ceramic, metal crown, and hard resin (plastic). The cost of implant placement surgery typically ranges from 100,000 to 200,000 yen, excluding hospitalization. The cost of the artificial tooth components depends on the connection method and type of abutment, as mentioned above, but generally ranges from 150,000 to 200,000 yen. Additionally, many dental clinics charge a fixed amount per tooth, with the total cost generally ranging from 300,000 to 400,000 yen.

For cleft lip and palate patients, the cost may be around 300,000 yen, as hospitalization is often required. The bone graft, which is sometimes necessary, may be covered by health insurance or may require out-of-pocket payment, depending on whether or not you plan to have an implant. It is essential to consult with your doctor to clarify this.

You may often come across advertisements such as "starting at 100,000 yen per implant," but the cost can vary significantly based on the manufacturer of the implant, the connection method, and the type of abutment used. Therefore, it is crucial to listen carefully to the explanations provided by the dental clinic.

Q What are the advantages and disadvantages?

Implant treatment has now been available for cleft lip and palate patients for about 10 years. Prior to that, dentures or bridge treatments were commonly used. Many cleft lip and palate patients have had bone grafts placed in the affected area, and there are some concerns regarding the long-term satisfaction with implant placement in the grafted bone.

Recently, most cases have progressed smoothly, but in rare instances, the grafted bone or implant may fail. With the introduction of implant treatment, the available options now include dentures, bridges, and implants. Let's compare the advantages and disadvantages of each.

A Advantages and disadvantages of dentures (Fig. 2)

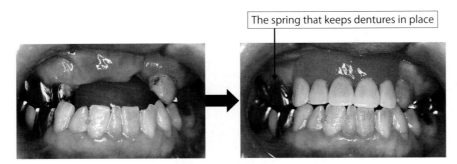

Fig. 2 Dentures

Advantages
- There is no need to grind down remaining teeth.
- Dentures are removable, making cleaning easier.
- If dentures no longer fit or break, repairs or remakes are relatively simple.
- They are relatively easy to fabricate.

Disadvantages
- The springs that hold the denture in place are visible, which limits esthetics.
- There may be psychological discomfort associated with wearing or removing dentures.
- Many cleft lip and palate patients are in their late teens to twenties, an age where self-consciousness is heightened, so it is important to consider this aspect carefully.

A Advantages and disadvantages of bridges (Fig. 3)

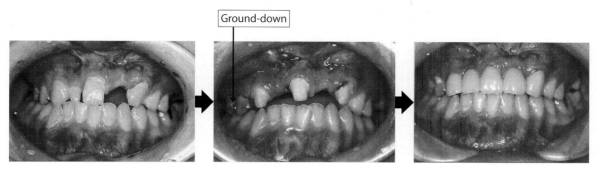

Fig. 3 Bridge

Advantages
- As a fixed restoration, bridges do not need to be removed like dentures.
- Bridges offer a natural appearance, blending well with the surrounding teeth.

Disadvantages
- Multiple adjacent teeth may need to be ground down to support the bridge.
- In some cases, the dental pulp (nerve) of the supporting teeth may need to be removed during the procedure.
- Since bridges are fixed, cleaning between and around the teeth can be challenging.
- Repairs and remanufacturing of bridges can be more complicated than other options.

A Advantages and disadvantages of implants (Fig. 4, 5)

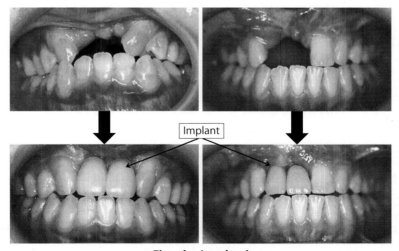

Fig. 4 Implant

CHAPTER 3. ORTHODONTICS, PROSTHODONTICS

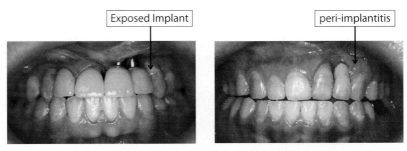

Fig. 5 Implant exposure and peri-implantitis

Advantages
- No need to grind down the surrounding teeth.
- Natural appearance.

Disadvantages
- Surgical treatment is required, and in some cases, hospitalization may be necessary.
- The financial burden is significant.
- Over time, there is a risk of gingival recession and peri-implantitis (periodontal disease around the implant), which can lead to the implant becoming exposed, loose, or even lost.
- Repairs and remanufacturing can be complex.

As mentioned, each method has its own advantages and disadvantages, so it is important to consult with your doctor.

Please discuss this thoroughly with your doctor and ensure you are fully satisfied before proceeding with treatment.

Q What is the limit on the duration of implant use?

A Implants do not have an expiration date.

However, age-related changes, such as bone resorption, can result in implant exposure. If the area around the implant is not kept clean, it can lead to periodontal disease, causing the gums to swell and bleed. In implants, this condition is referred to as peri-implantitis. If left untreated, peri-implantitis can progress, causing the implant to loosen, fail, or break. If untreated, the implant may eventually loosen and fall out. This progression is similar to what occurs with natural teeth affected by periodontal disease.

To ensure long-term use of implants, regular maintenance and follow-up care are essential. Maintenance typically includes radiographic evaluations (e.g., X-rays) to assess the condition of the implant body and surrounding bone. This is especially important for implants placed in grafted bone, requiring periodic radiographic monitoring. Regular maintenance appointments, which may be scheduled once every 3 months or once every 6 months or once a year, focus on:
- Plaque and calculus (tartar) assessment and removal.
- Oral hygiene guidance, including brushing techniques.
- Evaluation of occlusion (bite alignment).

Over time, the abutment (crown or artificial tooth components) may wear down or fracture. This wear and tear are also comparable to what occurs with natural teeth.

Discuss the appropriate frequency of maintenance visits with your provider based on the condition of your implant. For cleft lip and palate patients, specific considerations may apply, so individualized guidance is crucial.

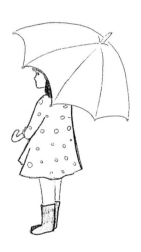

CHAPTER 3. ORTHODONTICS, PROSTHODONTICS

[Q] 61. HOW SHOULD I PROCEED IF I NEED TO CHANGE ORTHODONTIC CLINICS DUE TO A TRANSFER? WHAT WILL HAPPEN TO THE TREATMENT COSTS UP UNTIL THAT POINT AND THE FUTURE COSTS?

[A] **If relocation makes it difficult to continue attending your current clinic, you should first verify if the new clinic is accredited as a designated medical institution for self-supporting medical care (self-reliance support), and assess the continuity of care with oral and maxillofacial surgery (OMFS). It is essential to consult with your current orthodontist or oral surgeon at the earliest opportunity.**

The cost of general orthodontic treatment is typically categorized as "private treatment" (out-of-pocket treatment), meaning that the full treatment cost is borne by the patient. The payment methods vary by clinic, but in many cases, the total cost for the orthodontic treatment, covering the period until the alignment of the permanent teeth is corrected, is paid in full at the early stages of treatment. If a refund of treatment costs is necessary, the progress of the treatment to that point will be taken into account, and the remaining balance will be refunded. Additionally, because treatment costs for private care vary by region and clinic, the refunded amount may not cover continued treatment at the new clinic, and if treatment is spread across multiple clinics, additional costs may arise.

However, in the case of orthodontic treatment for cleft lip and palate, health insurance can be applied. Health insurance coverage will be based on the medical services provided on the day of the treatment.

The patient is required to pay the out-of-pocket portion of the treatment costs at the clinic on the day of the visit. Therefore, there will be no refund for the treatment costs incurred up until the move, as these costs correspond to the orthodontic treatment services provided up to that point. After the relocation, the cost of treatment, if covered by health insurance, will not differ significantly by region within Japan, as health insurance provides a standard rate across the country, unlike private treatment, where costs may vary. The patient will continue to pay the out-of-pocket portion for each procedure at the new clinic, just as they did at the previous one.

However, if the patient is receiving financial assistance through programs like medical care, it is important to note that the new clinic must be a designated rehabilitation medical institution. Therefore, when transferring orthodontic treatment due to relocation, it is advised to consult with the current orthodontist, who can refer the patient to a nearby designated medical institution.

Additionally, to ensure a smooth continuation of orthodontic treatment and proper handover to the new dentist, it is necessary to prepare and provide transfer documents, including information on the initial occlusion, the treatment history, and the planned course of future treatment, to the new orthodontist.

    In any case, if relocating makes it difficult to continue treatment at the current hospital, it is crucial to consult the attending orthodontist or oral surgeon early, as there may be a relationship between orthodontic treatment and oral surgery.

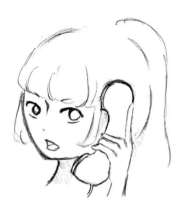

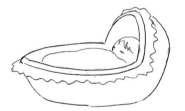

CHAPTER *4.* SPEECH, LANGUAGE

CHAPTER 4. SPEECH, LANGUAGE

[Q] 62. PLEASE TELL ME ABOUT DEVELOPMENTAL AND PSYCHOLOGICAL TESTS

[A] **These are assessments conducted to evaluate intellectual development and aptitudes, particularly in children with cleft lip and/or palate (CL/P). The tests may involve face-to-face interactions between the examiner and the child, interviews with parents to gather detailed insights, or questionnaire formats completed by the parents themselves. These assessments are crucial for understanding potential developmental challenges and tailoring support for children with CL/P.**

Developmental and psychological tests are used to assess a child's growth and abilities, including their intelligence, aptitude, and personality. These tests help in understanding the child's development and identifying any areas where they may need extra support, which can guide appropriate treatment or care. While cleft lip and palate itself does not cause developmental delays, these tests can help ensure that your child is growing and developing in a healthy way. Some tests involve direct interaction between the examiner and your child, where they may answer questions, solve mazes, or complete drawing tasks.

Other tests may involve an interview with the parents or be in the form of a questionnaire that you, as the parents, fill out. There are different types of tests, including developmental tests and intelligence tests. Some tests provide results in terms of an intelligence quotient (IQ), while others give a developmental quotient or measure the child's developmental age.

These tests require specialized knowledge and training to conduct and interpret. It's important not to be overly concerned about the specific numbers or scores, but instead to see the results as a way to gain insight into one part of your child's development. These tests can help the healthcare team understand your child better and offer the most suitable care based on their individual needs.

92

Specific examples of tests for children

Test name	Target age	Content
Enjoji-style Infant and Child Developmental Analysis Test	0 months to 4 years 8 months old	Question survey for parents Examines motor skill, social interaction and language development
Child Mental Developmental Diagnostic Test	0 to 7 years old	Question survey for parents Examines the development of each area: motor, cognition, social lifestyle, eating habit and language
New K-type Development Test	0 to 14 years	Direct testing Determining developmental age, developmental index and profile
Tanaka-Bine Intelligence Test	2 years old till adult	Direct testing Determining intelligence quotient (IQ) and mental age
WPPSI Intelligence Diagnostic Test	3 years and 10 months - 7 years 1month old	Direct testing Calculate intelligence quotient (IQ)

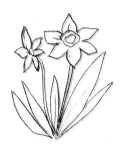

CHAPTER 4. SPEECH, LANGUAGE

[Q] 63. FOR CHILDREN WITH A CLEFT LIP, IS THERE A POSSIBILITY OF SPEECH OR LANGUAGE DISORDERS?

[A] **Following cleft lip repair surgery, the closure and function of the lip are typically restored to a level where significant impairment is unlikely. Therefore, it is generally considered that a cleft lip would not adversely affect speech articulation or phonation after surgical intervention.**

Children with cleft lip typically do not experience significant issues with speech after surgery, as the surgery helps close the lip and allows normal lip movement. This means that cleft lip itself does not usually affect pronunciation. However, it is important to understand how speech works.

When we speak, we make sounds by adjusting the shape of our mouth and using our lips, tongue, and breath. For example, vowels like "a," "i," and "u" are made by opening the mouth, while consonants like "p," "b," and "m" are produced by closing the lips.

In children with cleft lip, sometimes there may be issues with producing the correct sounds, especially those that involve the lips, such as "f" and "w." While cleft lip surgery usually helps with lip movement, it's a good idea to check your child's speech development once they start kindergarten or school. A speech and pronunciation test may help identify any issues with pronunciation or language development, especially related to jaw or lip function.

Some sounds in speech are produced with the breath moving through the mouth while the tongue changes its position, and in some cases, a speech-language therapist may be needed if the cleft affects speech further. This situation is rare, though, and most speech sounds are made with the exhalation of breath.

In general, cleft lip surgery helps restore the ability to produce sounds with the correct airflow through the mouth, and as the child grows, they should be able to make most sounds properly. It's important to remember that language and pronunciation are skills that develop over time, and speech issues can often be addressed with therapy and practice.

Q 64. IF THE SURGERY FOR CLEFT LIP IS DELAYED, WILL IT AFFECT SPEECH AND LANGUAGE?

A Environmental factors, such as delayed surgery, may influence the development of language.

Cleft lip repair surgery is typically performed when the baby weighs less than 6 kg and is 3 months old. If the weight is insufficient or if there are other comorbid conditions, the surgery may be delayed.

For children with a cleft palate, there is a significant risk of speech development being affected due to the structural issues of the mouth. However, for children with only a cleft lip, the impact on speech is generally minimal. Nevertheless, if surgery is delayed and hospitalization results in limited interaction with others, it can negatively influence language development.

The key is ensuring that communication skills develop well. It is important to engage the child with frequent verbal interactions and actively encourage communication from those around them.

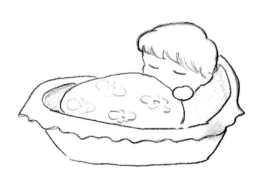

CHAPTER 4. SPEECH, LANGUAGE

[Q] 65. IF A CHILD WITH A CLEFT PALATE IS DELAYED IN RECEIVING SURGERY DUE TO LOW WEIGHT, WILL IT AFFECT THEIR LANGUAGE OR ACADEMIC DEVELOPMENT IN THE FUTURE?

[A] **It is important for a speech-language pathologist to explain the child's vocal and language characteristics, and for the adults around the child to provide appropriate support and encouragement. Such interventions can have a significant impact on the child's future language development.**

When performing surgery, ensuring overall stability and securing physiological functions is of primary importance. The timing of surgery may be delayed depending on the child's weight or the presence of comorbidities, in addition to the cleft palate.

For children with a cleft palate, the oral and nasal cavities are connected, which creates an unfavorable environment for feeding, drinking, and articulating speech sounds. To improve this environment, a palatal obturator or prosthetic device may be used to temporarily separate the oral and nasal cavities. However, this is a temporary solution and does not replicate the surgical repair of the velum (soft palate) or the hard palate.

The child's oral environment will not be identical to that after the reconstructive surgery of the cleft palate, but the palatal obturator can facilitate feeding and allow for the production of a variety of speech sounds.

It is essential that a speech-language pathologist (SLP) intervene early to support the child's speech and language development, even before surgery. Children do not begin acquiring speech only after surgery; they start internalizing the language and sounds they hear from caregivers, even with compromised oral conditions.

A speech-language pathologist should assess the child's speech and language characteristics, and caregivers should provide appropriate, consistent support. Early intervention, such as speech stimulation and auditory exposure, will significantly influence the child's future speech and language development.

Q 66. DO CHILDREN NEED SPEECH THERAPY AFTER CLEFT PALATE SURGERY?

A **In some cases, speech therapy may be needed. It is recommended to regularly monitor the child's speech articulation.**

Cleft palate surgery is typically performed around the age of 18 months, taking into account both maxillary development and language acquisition. The primary goal of surgery during this period is to close the oral cavity, thereby promoting healthy speech development as the child begins to speak. When surgery is performed at the appropriate time, and adequate closure of the oral cavity is achieved, some children may naturally acquire normal speech without the need for special training.

However, even after achieving proper oral closure, some children may continue to exhibit abnormal speech patterns due to ingrained habits. In such cases, speech therapy may be necessary to correct these speech patterns. Even if speech has improved somewhat, slight inaccuracies may remain, and these should also be addressed.

Additionally, in some cases, despite surgical intervention, the muscle movement of the soft palate may still be insufficient. In these instances, training to enhance the movement of the soft palate and facilitate proper oral closure is essential.

Training typically starts with exercises to strengthen oral closure and practice exhalation through the mouth. Monitoring for nasal airflow during exhalation helps assess the oral cavity's state. Once the child can exhale forcefully through the mouth, the next step is to correct each abnormal speech sound. The specific sounds to be corrected will be determined based on the child's individual speech patterns. The goal of therapy is to return all speech sounds to normal.

Even after cleft palate surgery, it is recommended to regularly monitor the child's speech articulation. Early detection of abnormal speech patterns allows for timely correction. As the child grows, changes in jaw structure may also influence speech, so if concerns arise, it is advisable to consult with speech therapist.

Reference

1) Takahashi S. Cleft Lip and Cleft Palate: Basics and Clinical Applications. Hyoron Publishers, Tokyo, 1996.

CHAPTER 4. SPEECH, LANGUAGE

[Q] 67. PLEASE ADVISE ON WHAT TO BE MINDFUL OF REGARDING LANGUAGE AT HOME BEFORE THE SURGERY

[A] Do not make the child repeat words or attempt to correct their pronunciation.

Children with clefts often speak with the intention of being correct, so if they are repeatedly corrected or asked to rephrase their speech, it may cause anxiety or a loss of confidence, leading to psychological issues.

Until speech therapy begins, avoid correcting their speech. Allow the child to speak freely and enjoy conversation in a relaxed, fun environment. Listen attentively to what the child says and accept their attempts. This interaction helps promote the development of the child's communication skills and language comprehension.

It is important not to treat the child with a cleft palate as different or special, but to raise them in a typical environment.

If needed, a speech-language pathologist will provide guidance at the appropriate time, so please follow their advice.

[Q] 68. YOU WERE ADVISED NOT TO CORRECT THE PRONUNCIATION, BUT WHY IS THAT?

[A] Forcing correction can lead to psychological issues such as anxiety or loss of confidence, and may even result in the child developing incorrect pronunciation.

After cleft palate surgery, the child may not yet have acquired proper velopharyngeal closure (the function where the soft palate elevates and contacts the pharyngeal wall to separate the oral and nasal cavities). During this period, speech may be unclear. While many children naturally develop normal pronunciation once velopharyngeal function is achieved, there are cases where unclear speech persists. In such cases, speech therapy will be necessary.

The cause of unclear speech can vary depending on the child. It may be related to age-related developmental delays or velopharyngeal insufficiency, which can occur if the soft palate does not function adequately. In these cases, additional interventions such as palatal surgery or the use of speech aids may be required. A speech-language pathologist will assess whether there are issues with

98

these functions and proceed with appropriate therapy.

Speech therapy typically begins around 4 to 5 years of age, but parents should refrain from forcing the child to correct their speech during this stage. Forcing correction may lead to psychological issues, such as the child avoiding speech due to the pressure of being told their speech is wrong, even when they believe it to be correct. Additionally, forced correction may result in the child learning an incorrect pronunciation.

Until therapy begins and speech pathologists provide guidance on home practice, parents should avoid making the child repeat words or correct their speech.

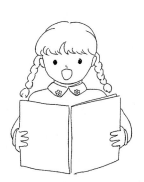

CHAPTER 4. SPEECH, LANGUAGE

[Q] 69. AFTER CLEFT PALATE SURGERY, IS THERE ANY TRAINING THAT CAN BE DONE AT HOME?

[A] Yes, there are language training activities that can be done at home after cleft palate surgery.

After cleft palate surgery, specialized treatment and management, including language therapy, are provided by professionals such as oral surgeons, pediatricians, ENT specialists, and speech-language pathologists. During this time, home-based interventions and language training tailored to the child's condition are known to enhance treatment outcomes and language development.

However, the language training programs conducted at home need to follow a precise plan devised by the attending specialists. Some families, out of eagerness, may try to implement their own methods of language training or spend several hours a day on therapy, leading to fatigue for both the parents and the child. This can disrupt the family's normal routine. Such actions usually stem from the parents' deep concern and high expectations for their child's growth and future. However, overdoing it can have adverse effects.

Excessive efforts in language training can have negative consequences, so caution is necessary. When carrying out home-based language training programs, it is important to follow the instructions provided by the attending physician. It is recommended to report the results of the training and any impacts on your child's daily routine, such as improvements in drinking from a straw of a certain size, to the speech-language pathologist for ongoing evaluation.

If families have difficulty to allocate time for language therapy at home

It is important to remember that the home environment is the foundation of a child's development, and worrying about such matters should be avoided. A stable home environment is crucial for the growth of a child. If parents become overly concerned about not having time for language training at home, it can negatively affect their ability to fulfill their parental role, which may, in turn, become an issue for the child's development.

However, when language training is needed for children with language impairments associated with cleft lip and palate, it is essential to seek professional guidance without hesitation. The healthcare provider will carefully consider the family's circumstances and collaborate to develop the best approach for the child's needs.

Q 70. MY CHILD HAS A HOLE AFTER CLEFT PALATE SURGERY. WILL THIS AFFECT THEIR SPEECH IN THE FUTURE?

A Just because there is a residual hole (fistula), it does not necessarily cause speech articulation issues.

Depending on the size and location of the opening (fistula), it may affect the voice and speech articulation. For example, the voice may sound nasal, with air escaping through the nose, resulting in a soft speech pattern. Alternatively, speaking from the back of the mouth could make the 'ta' sounds resemble 'ka' sounds. However, just because there is a fistula, it does not necessarily cause speech problems.

If the fistula is affecting the articulation or voice, using a fistula closure prosthesis (palatal obturator) may significantly improve these issues.

Cleft palate treatment begins with surgical intervention in infancy and continues throughout adulthood, so the treatment priorities may change over time. To determine if the fistula is affecting speech, a proper speech and language evaluation by a speech-language pathologist is recommended. If it is impacting speech, please consult with your physician to select the appropriate treatment plan in alignment with your child's ongoing care.

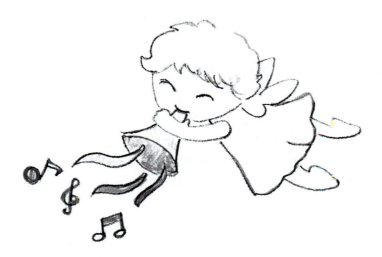

CHAPTER 4. SPEECH, LANGUAGE

[Q] 71. PLEASE LET ME KNOW ABOUT SPEECH AND LANGUAGE TRAINING

[A] **There are various methods of speech therapy, so please refer to the following.**

Training on how to make sounds

Speech therapy is generally provided by speech-language pathologists (SLP), who work in hospitals or speech therapy classrooms at speech-language pathology training schools. From the time children first begin to speak, parents closely observe their children's progress in communication. While there are individual differences in children's development, there are times when parents may feel concerned about their child's speech progress.

First, concerns are addressed by discussing the details, or the SLP may directly interview the child to assess their speech patterns. If a child's speech is unclear to the listener, the SLP will investigate the way each sound is produced. For example, when trying to pronounce certain sounds, the child may produce another sound, or some sounds may not be pronounced clearly. These speech errors are addressed through practice, and the child gradually learns how to produce the correct sounds. If therapy with the SLP is recommended, a schedule is made after consulting with the family.

Each speech sound has a specific manner of production, such as which parts of the mouth are involved. For instance, the "pa" and "ma" sounds are produced using the lips. The "pa" sound involves closing the lips and then releasing air to create the sound. The SLP breaks down the motion needed to produce each sound into smaller steps and demonstrates them in a way that is easy for the child to understand. For example, blowing air toward a small piece of paper helps practice the "pa" or "pi" sounds.

The process of producing speech sounds is broken into small steps. Since these steps are small, the process may take time, but the general principle is that smaller steps are easier to manage. Learning to produce one sound leads to word formation, reading books, and eventually holding conversations.

The shape and function of the mouth can influence the production of speech sounds. In children with cleft lip and palate, the shape and function of the oral structures can affect how sounds are produced. As treatment through surgery or orthodontics is carried out in collaboration with other specialists, speech therapy for the child can continue to help with correct sound production.

Effect of straw practice

Straw practice involves placing a straw in a glass of water and blowing to create bubbles. The primary focus of this practice is to engage the movement of the soft palate (uvula) and surrounding areas. When someone says "ah," you can observe that the uvula area moves upwards, which is a sign of the soft palate's motion. The purpose of using the straw to blow water is to replicate this

102

movement.

In speech production, it is necessary to push air from the lungs into the mouth. As air passes between the tongue and teeth, it forms the sounds of speech, and air vibrating the vocal cords is needed for producing voice. Thus, blowing through the straw mimics the action of expelling air from the mouth and activating the soft palate area, which prevents air from escaping through the nose. Conversely, when speaking or singing with a resonant sound, air is allowed to pass through the nasal cavity. The muscles around the soft palate contract, closing off the airflow to the nose, similar to the way a camera shutter closes after it has opened.

During speech, eating, or playing an instrument like a trumpet, the closure of the nasal airway is necessary. During swallowing or trumpet playing, the closure is stronger, as the breath is forceful. In comparison, the airflow and nasal closure during speech are less forceful. By blowing water through a straw, the movement of the soft palate is trained in a way that resembles speech production, reinforcing the closure of the nasal passage.

Effect of gargling practice

Gargling can be used to practice sounds like "ka" and "ga." When gargling, individuals naturally produce the sound "gagaga" without even thinking about it. Even if a child has difficulty pronouncing "ka" or "ga," the act of gargling helps to initiate the production of the "ga" sound. Once the child is able to produce the "ga" sound, further structured practice may be needed for them to incorporate it naturally into conversation.

When gargling, the head is tilted back, and water collects in the back of the mouth. To prevent water from entering the throat, the tongue rises to the roof of the mouth, blocking the water. Though we may not consciously feel the tongue doing this, the water would enter the throat if the tongue didn't block it. This action of raising the tongue to the roof of the mouth also occurs when producing the "ka" or "ga" sounds. Thus, gargling practice serves as a foundation for speech sound production. When the tongue releases the blocked air, it produces the sound "ga" or "ka". Through consistent practice with each sound, the child can gradually improve their pronunciation.

Speech practice is an important first step. This type of practice method has been developed through various trial and error over time and is the result of efforts made to make it practical. Researchers studied how speech sounds are articulated and created methods to convey the process in a way that is easy to understand for those learning. These methods were designed to break down speech sounds into manageable steps for effective learning and are the result of constant refinement and thought by those dedicated to the field.

Orthodontic appliances, made of metal, often make contact with the roof of the mouth, which may create frequent discomfort for the tongue. When orthodontic treatment is undertaken and the oral environment improves, issues with speech sounds, which were previously noticeable, may disappear. This is because the alignment of the teeth and the shape of the upper jaw can directly affect speech sounds. It is important to monitor for any new speech issues, such as excessive nasality, which may arise while speaking (although nasality issues are generally not directly related to orthodontics, it is still important to pay attention to them).

As the growth of the jaw and pharynx stabilizes, and orthodontic treatment is completed, monitoring speech progress during middle and high school years can sometimes be done at a local speech therapy center rather than at the original hospital, to help reduce the burden of regular visits.

Reference

1) Ogata Y. Speech Language Hearing Therapy Series 8: Organic Speech Disorders. edited by Saito H. 8th ed. Kenpaku-sha, Tokyo, 2010, 130, 132.

Orthodontic appliances and speech therapy

Wearing orthodontic appliances can lead to discomfort or difficulties in speech, as these devices may alter the positioning of teeth and affect speech clarity. Some appliances are used to correct the alignment of teeth, while others aim to promote the growth of the upper jaw. In some cases, the narrowing of the mouth caused by these devices can impact speech production. Therefore, even while undergoing orthodontic treatment, it is necessary to monitor speech performance and continue observing any speech issues that arise.

When orthodontic treatment begins, especially after the start of elementary school, the majority of articulation training should already be completed. If articulation practice is nearly finished, there is no need to spend extensive time on speech training. Instead, it is sufficient to attend speech therapy sessions once or twice a year to monitor progress. The monitoring period should continue, as bodily growth, along with changes in the shape of the mouth and pharynx, can affect speech production. Changes related to how air passes through the nose during speech should also be carefully observed.

Remote speech and language training

For individuals who live far from speech therapy centers, remote speech therapy (tele practice) is an effective option. This method allows patients to continue speech therapy with a speech-language pathologist, even if they are living abroad, as if they were attending in-person sessions. This reduces the burden of travel and allows for more frequent sessions. As a result, therapy sessions can be more consistent, helping to improve therapy outcomes without the fatigue associated with travel.

Training can be conducted in a relaxed home environment. The materials used include a computer, a web camera, and the internet via Skype. These are all commercially available products, so they are not specialized equipment and are easily accessible. However, there are no insurance-covered settings for this. It is provided as a private treatment or partially for free as a social service, so confirmation is necessary.

In speech training, speech-language therapists need to accurately listen to the patient's pronunciation. The patient must receive proper guidance because of this reason. Non-linguistic ability development refers to different things from pronunciation training. Specifically, it involves developing abilities that are earlier than pronunciation training. The foundation for speech pronunciation is considered to be language development. This training aims to enrich those aspects. The training uses various educational materials. For example, there are large picture cards and toys that roll, fly, or bounce. One significant feature of this training is that it involves content that is enjoyable for children. It can also be done in various settings, including online.

The materials are offered in various ways from the side conducting the training. On the patient's computer screen, the speech-language therapist's image appears, and on the therapist's computer, the patient's condition appears, and the speech training is conducted through sound and images. It has already been verified whether this can be done through voice and images over the internet. The results from such training can match the outcomes of traditional face-to-face speech training. This ability development is called communicative behavior. There is a growing movement to actively promote this kind of foundational ability development. Children absorb stimulating activities in a fun and playful atmosphere. They are encouraged to receive stimuli that promote growth at the stage of their development, preparing them for future growth.

Non-linguistic skill development

Traditional speech training involves visits to the hospital, but it has already been verified whether this can be done through online speech therapy. Speech training typically starts from around ages 4 to 5. By this age, children can hear almost all the sounds in the Japanese language, and they can begin to acquire sounds. The development of language and communication abilities is encouraged, which is why it's called an early intervention program. There's nothing particularly difficult about it. The daily interactions that parents have with their children provide various stimuli that promote the child's growth. A parent's smile, moving their child's arms and legs, or using fingers to grab something — these activities encourage the child's growth using all five senses. Even in traditional speech pronunciation training, children do not talk directly to the speech-language therapist from the beginning, so toys like animated dolls are used to engage the children's interest. Through these interactions, the sounds that emerge are gradually expanded into words and sentences. Efforts to work with children from an early stage have already started.

Contact Information:

Aichi Gakuin University Hospital, Speech Therapy Outpatient Department

052-751-7181 (Ext.) 5223

Reference

1) Ogata Y. Speech Language Hearing Therapy Series 8: Organic Speech Disorders. edited by Saito H. 8th ed. Kenpaku-sha, Tokyo, 2010, 120.

CHAPTER 4. SPEECH, LANGUAGE

Q 72. WHAT IS VELOPHARYNGEAL DYSFUNCTION?

A It is when the oral cavity and nasal cavity cannot be properly separated, causing air to escape through the nose.

The oral and nasal cavities are connected at the throat, and the movement of the soft palate (the posterior part of the roof of the mouth, including the uvula) regulates their opening and closing. When breathing through the nose, the soft palate lowers, allowing air to pass through the nose. On the other hand, when speaking or swallowing, the soft palate rises, blocking the passage to the nasal cavity. This function is known as velopharyngeal closure function.

In the case of cleft palate, the separation between the oral and nasal cavities is not properly achieved, leading to the possibility of velopharyngeal dysfunction, where air escapes through the nose (refer to the diagram below). Even after surgery, if the length or movement of the soft palate is insufficient, velopharyngeal dysfunction may persist. As a result, problems such as nasal voice or difficulty pronouncing words may occur when speaking.

To assess velopharyngeal closure function, tests such as placing a specialized mirror under the nostrils to check for nasal airflow, voice quality and pronunciation evaluations, X-ray imaging, and endoscopic examinations are performed. Additionally, exercises such as blowing a trumpet or straw may be recommended to improve nasal-oral separation and achieve optimal velopharyngeal closure function.

Q 73. PLEASE TELL ME ABOUT HYPERNASALITY

A In many cases, hypernasality is simply a phenomenon caused by velopharyngeal dysfunction or palatal fistula.

Hypernasality refers to a voice that is overly resonant in the nasal cavity. However, it differs from the "nasal voice" that occurs when your nose is blocked due to crying after watching a movie or having a cold. The nasal voice in such cases is referred to as hyponasal voice, which is the "opposite" of hypernasality.

Hypernasality occurs when the vowels excessively resonate in the nasal cavity. It is usually caused by velopharyngeal dysfunction. A large palatal fistula or an unrepaired cleft palate can also contribute.

When speaking, the soft palate (the muscle near the uvula) normally rises to prevent exhaled air from entering the nose. However, in cases of velopharyngeal dysfunction, this air flows into the nasal cavity, causing resonance and producing a hypernasal sound. In the case of a large fistula or an unrepaired area in the palate, the airflow from the mouth to the nose can pass through the opening and resonate, leading to hypernasality.

The presence of hypernasality does not directly cause difficulty in articulation, nor does it cause sounds like a strained "a" (glottal stop) or "ma" (distorted consonants due to nasal airflow). In most cases, hypernasality is a phenomenon caused by velopharyngeal dysfunction or palatal fistula.

There are various reasons why speech may not be produced correctly, but it can be clearly stated that hypernasality is not the cause. However, if hypernasality is present, its cause needs to be identified, and careful monitoring of the child's development is essential. Even if there are no articulation errors, detailed, periodic follow-up from the cleft palate treatment team is necessary to ensure proper speech development.

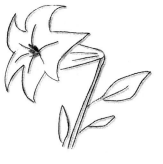

CHAPTER 4. SPEECH, LANGUAGE

Q 74. WHAT IS ABNORMAL ARTICULATION?

A **Articulation refers to pronunciation, and abnormal articulation refers to pronunciations that are not typically observed in normal development. Examples of typical abnormal articulation include nasal speech (also known as nasalized articulation), palatalized articulation, lateralized articulation, and glottal stop sounds.**

Here are examples of each abnormal articulation.

Nasal resonance articulation

In the area where sounds are produced using the mouth and tongue, the tongue closes the mouth, and the sound is created in the nasal cavity, resulting in a "kunkun" sound.

Palatalized articulation

The pronunciation is distorted because air is exhaled through the mouth.
The tongue's tip and the upper front teeth create a sound like "ta-da."

Glottal stop sound

This sound is produced by forcefully closing the vocal cords or false vocal cords in the larynx, causing the breath to be temporarily blocked.

Speech errors in normal development

In the typical developmental process, vowels appear by age 1, consonants by age 1, and all sounds begin to emerge by age 4-6. As seen above, up until about the age of 3 everyone makes mistakes in pronunciation. Errors such as substituting "okasan" (mother) with "otaa-san" (substitution), "kuruma" (car) with "kuru" (assimilation), or "sakana" (fish) with "sana" (assimilation) are common and do not fall under abnormal articulation. In such cases, unlike abnormal articulation, language instruction is generally not actively provided until after **4 years old**, and it is desirable to observe the progress with specialists.

Cleft lip and palate speech development

By **6 years old**, the pronunciation of "ta-da" and similar sounds will be produced in the same way as adults, as the structure and function of the mouth from the cleft lip and palate become normal.

Palatalization

The tongue moves toward the back of the mouth and replaces or distorts sounds such as "ka-ga" or "hi."

108

Lateralization of articulation

Normally, air is expelled through the central part of the mouth (from the front), but when the lower jaw or tongue moves to the side, lateral speech errors occur.

Mispronunciations due to structural issues

These are typically caused by conditions like cleft lip and palate where pronunciation may be unclear. These issues are referred to as "organic articulation disorders" and require long-term specialized treatment and planning by experts. SLP training is required.

Q 75. WHAT CAN BE UNDERSTOOD FROM A FIBER SCOPE EXAMINATION?

A **A fiber scope examination allows to directly observe the movement of the soft palate and pharynx, which cannot be determined by an X-ray examination alone. It is a very useful method for understanding the current state of various pronunciations, blowing, swallowing, and other functions.**

One of the disabilities in patients with cleft palate is nasopharyngeal closure dysfunction. Nasopharyngeal closure refers to the closure of the passage between the mouth and nose. The examination methods for nasopharyngeal closure function include blowing tests, nasal airflow mirror tests, X-ray examinations, fiber scope (endoscopic) examinations, and other methods. These examinations help understand the current state, such as whether the speech disorder is related to nasopharyngeal closure dysfunction or not, and determine what kind of training should be provided.

The fiber scope examination is very useful for understanding the current state of various pronunciations, blowing, swallowing, and other functions that cannot be fully determined by X-ray alone.

The nasopharyngeal closure function is essential for closing the air passage at the soft palate and pharynx for speaking and blowing air from the mouth. If this function doesn't work well, it can lead to problems like nasal voice, speech disorders, and difficulties in inflating a balloon or playing a recorder. Language evaluation is necessary, and if there are speech disorders, it is important to address them.

The fiber scope examination involves applying anesthetic to the nasal cavity (with a cotton swab or similar) and inserting the fiber scope through the nostrils to observe the upper part of the soft palate. This examination method is very useful for observing the movements of the soft palate and pharynx, which cannot be determined by other methods, allowing us to assess the current state of various functions such as speech, blowing, and swallowing. This test is generally painless and can

109

be performed on children as young as around 6 years old, with over 95% of children being able to undergo this procedure.

The nasopharyngeal closure function is important in determining whether it is working well, whether it can completely close during blowing and swallowing, and if the closure is weak, what movements should be made to improve closure. By observing these factors, it is possible to apply this information to language therapy. Furthermore, if language training alone seems to improve the condition, it is important to consider whether it would be better to use speech aids or other pronunciation assistive devices for training.

Even if the speech language is currently good, it is crucial to monitor the age-related changes in the width of the nasopharynx, the size of the adenoids, and the changes in the movement of the soft palate and pharynx for nasopharyngeal closure. Observing these changes is essential for ongoing monitoring. Therefore, fiber scope examinations at our facility are typically conducted at the following stages:

1. Initial assessment of nasopharyngeal closure function
2. Second growth phase
3. Long-term follow-up observation

During this period, the adenoids begin to regress, and if there is any dysfunction in nasopharyngeal closure, it is important to assess the situation promptly and provide training to recover function, as recovery is easier at this early stage, which helps prevent further deterioration.

For cleft palate patients who have undergone the initial surgery and language therapy, over 90% of children recover their function. However, in about 5% of children, some speech disorders may still appear, and in such cases, a reassessment of the need for a second surgery might be necessary.

The fiber scope examination is an important tool for assessing these functions, and when using speech aids, it can help observe the nasopharynx to assess the effectiveness of the device or adjust the valve of the speech aid. It is also useful for postoperative observation and combined with language training, it helps monitor the progress after surgery.

Regular check-ups, including fiber scope examinations, are performed even if the evaluation is good. The second growth phase occurs during late elementary school to middle school age, when not only the body but also the motor and autonomic nervous systems are completing their final stages of development. Therefore, it is crucial to monitor the status of nasopharyngeal closure function during

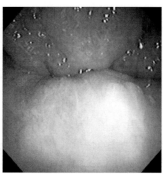
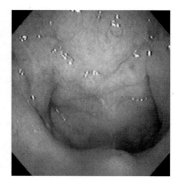

Endoscopic findings during pronunciation **Endoscopic findings at rest**

this period.

Even after a second surgery, some patients may still exhibit slight speech disorders. Oral surgeons, ENT specialists, plastic surgeons, and speech therapists work together to maximize the child's abilities and assist in the recovery of language function. The fiber scope examination is one of the tools used for this purpose.

[Q] 76. WHAT CAN BE DETERMINED FROM A CEPHALOMETRIC EXAMINATION?

[A] It helps identify the cause of malocclusion.

A cephalometric examination is a type of X-ray that helps doctors examine the bones and structure of the face, particularly the upper and lower jaw. It is often used to understand the cause of malocclusion, which is when the teeth do not align properly.

Unlike regular X-rays, cephalometric allows the orthodontist to accurately measure the size, position, and angle of the jaw bones. This detailed information helps the orthodontist create a personalized treatment plan, especially for children with clefts, who may need special care for jaw alignment and dental development.

By using cephalometric measurements along with dental models, the orthodontist can determine the best approach for correcting any issues with the bite, leading to better long-term results. This tool is essential for planning orthodontic treatments and ensuring the child's facial and dental development is on track.

[Q] 77. WHAT ARE SPEECH AIDS AND PALATAL LIFT PROSTHESES (PLP)? AND WHEN ARE THEY USED?

[A] These are devices that assist with nasal pharyngeal closure function. Both devices physically narrow the nasal pharyngeal cavity. Details are provided below.

Speech aids (**Fig. 1**) and palatal lift prostheses (PLP) (**Fig. 3**) are devices that assist with nasal pharyngeal closure function. After cleft palate surgery, if there is residual nasal speech or nasal pharyngeal closure dysfunction, these devices are used. The causes include "fistula in the palatal region" and "nasal pharyngeal closure dysfunction," which is associated with the movement of the

111

soft palate.

There are two main causes: one due to motor dysfunction and the other due to a wide nasal pharynx (short soft palate) (**Fig. 2**). For palatal fistulas, the fistula closure bed can also be used.

Speech aids are used to insert a plug (valve) into the nasal pharynx, which helps activate the movement of these muscles. Palatal lift prostheses (PLP) (**Fig. 3**) are used to elevate the soft palate and are primarily used for motor dysfunctions in the soft palate (**Fig. 4**). In cases where the soft palate is completely nonfunctional, these devices may not be effective. For a wide nasal pharynx (short soft palate), if the force is too strong, it may cause ulcers in the soft palate.

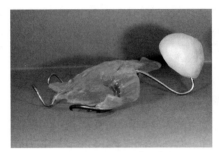

Fig. 1 Speech aid

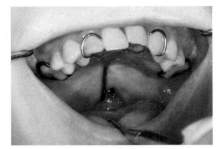

Fig. 2 When using a speech aid

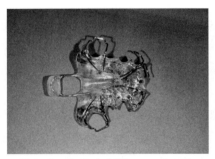

Fig. 3 Palatal lift prosthesis (PLP)

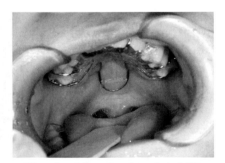

Fig. 4 Attached palatal lift prosthesis (PLP)

Both devices work by physically narrowing the nasal pharynx, but the palatal lift prosthesis (PLP) stimulates the soft palate and, additionally, muscles on the pharyngeal wall. The speech aid works similarly, but it involves adjusting the valve size to ensure that it can close during functional use and open slightly during resting periods. This requires careful adjustment.

If there are any issues or adjustments needed, especially with the speech aid, it is important to visit the facility that created the device.

[Q] 78. DOES SURGERY ON THE ADENOIDS AFFECT SPEECH?

[A] **Exudative otitis media caused by enlarged adenoids tends to lead to conductive hearing loss. If there are issues with hearing function, speech development may also be delayed as a result.**

Increased adenoids can cause otitis media with effusion, which tends to lead to conductive hearing loss, potentially causing problems with hearing function. The adenoids (pharyngeal tonsils) are lymphatic tissues located in the posterior upper part of the nasopharynx. After adenoidectomy, there can be nasopharyngeal closure dysfunction. Evaluation through radiographs and fiberoptic endoscopy is crucial. Adenoidectomy is common in children with cleft palates. However, there are individual differences, and after surgery, submucous clefts may appear in some cases. Although the condition of the nasopharyngeal closure can improve after adenoidectomy, in children who have undergone cleft lip and palate surgery, the adenoids may also shrink and regress over time.

The position of the adenoids plays a role in nasopharyngeal closure when speaking. During times when the adenoids are enlarged, contact between the soft palate and adenoid may contribute to good nasopharyngeal closure. However, if adenoids are removed, nasal voice or nasal leakage may suddenly appear, especially in cases where the soft palate is short or weak. In these cases, before performing adenoidectomy, specialist examination of the soft palate and hard palate should be performed to assess the risks and benefits.

When symptoms begin to appear, even children with cleft palates may experience delayed speech development due to the removal of adenoids. Therefore, a comprehensive assessment, including the prognosis after surgery, is necessary before proceeding with adenoidectomy.

In children with cleft palates, it is essential to conduct an evaluation before adenoidectomy to assess the relationship between the position of the adenoids and the nasopharyngeal closure site, the

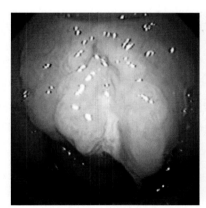

Photo taken by fiber optic endoscopy at rest when adenoids are involved in velopharyngeal closure

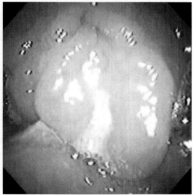

Photo taken by fiber optic endoscopy during pronunciation when adenoids are involved in velopharyngeal closure

CHAPTER 4. SPEECH, LANGUAGE

length and movement of the soft palate, and the depth (width) of the pharynx.

References

1) Kataura A. An Organ with Two Faces: Tonshils and Their Diseases. Nanzando, Tokyo, 2005.

2) Wada T. (ed.) Pathology, Diagnosis, and Treatment. Ishiyaku Publishers, Tokyo, 2005.

3) Tachimura T. Velar and Pharyngeal Closure Deficiency: Its Pathology, Diagnosis, and Treatment. Ishiyaku Publishers, Tokyo, 2012.

Q 79. IS IT POSSIBLE FOR PRONUNCIATION TO WORSEN AFTER ENTERING ELEMENTARY SCHOOL?

A **There is a possibility. There are various reasons for this, but one common cause is orthodontic treatment that often begins around the elementary school years.**

For instance, treatments like braces that help widen the jaw can sometimes make the hole in the upper jaw (the cleft) larger. This may cause the child's voice to sound more nasal, or lead to unclear speech. These braces can be placed on either the upper or lower jaw.

Before any orthodontic appliances are used, your child will need a thorough evaluation to determine if they are necessary. Your doctor or orthodontist will work with you to choose the right treatment. If the cleft opening becomes larger during treatment, there are options to help close it, and with proper care, your child can regain clear speech.

However, it's important to remember that ongoing support from a speech-language therapist is crucial. This will help prevent the child from developing bad speech habits while wearing braces.

You might notice changes like your child's speech becoming harder to understand, their voice sounding more nasal, or they might make sounds from the back of their nose when they speak. This can happen because of the braces. If the hole in the palate becomes wider, it's important to assess how much this is affecting their speech.

In most cases, any speech problems caused by orthodontic treatment are temporary. Once the braces are removed, speech often improves. However, as your child grows, the way they speak might change, and their cleft may need additional care. Regular evaluations by a speech-language therapist are essential, even if your child's speech seemed fine when they were younger. Therapy should continue until all treatments for the cleft palate are complete.

114

Q 80. IF THERE IS AN ABNORMALITY IN PRONUNCIATION, COULD IT BE DUE TO A CLEFT PALATE, EVEN IF THERE IS NO VISIBLE EXTERNAL ABNORMALITY?

A In cases of submucous cleft palate, there may be a split in the palatal muscles or bones, and the condition may also involve a cleft uvula.

Although no obvious cleft is seen and the palate may appear normal at first glance, there may be a split in the palatal muscles or bones under the mucous membrane, and a cleft uvula (commonly referred to as "the uvula") may also be present.

Submucous cleft palate, like a regular cleft palate, can lead to nasal cavity closure dysfunction, resulting in milk leakage from the nose, unclear speech, or speech disorders.

Unlike a visible cleft, the abnormality of the palate is often difficult to detect, which can delay diagnosis and lead to inappropriate treatment or language training without identifying the underlying cause. However, some individuals may have normal speech despite this condition.

Thus, even if diagnosed with submucous cleft palate, the choice of treatment—such as palate surgery, prosthetic treatment, and language training—depends on the individual case, with language assessment being crucial in determining the appropriate course of action.

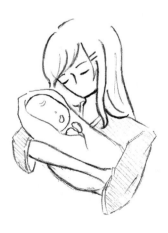

CHAPTER 4. SPEECH, LANGUAGE

[Q] 81. I AM STRUGGLING WITH HOW TO COMMUNICATE WITH MY SON, WHO WAS BORN WITH A CLEFT PALATE. AT ONE AND A HALF YEARS OLD, HE IS NOT SAYING ANY WORDS OTHER THAN "MAMA" AND IS COMMUNICATING THROUGH GESTURES AND SIGNS. WHAT SHOULD I DO?

[A] **It is very good that you are communicating through gestures and signs. If you are primarily using actions with minimal verbal communication, it would be beneficial to actively use voice and words as well. If there are delays in language comprehension or issues with social interactions and behavior, it is advisable to consult a professional institution for guidance.**

Using gestures and signs to communicate with your child is an excellent approach. Much of the information we process comes through our visual senses. Using signs and gestures likely enhances your child's understanding of words and situations, and it's commendable that you've started this approach naturally or with thoughtful planning. You are likely combining these gestures with verbal communication effectively. If, however, you are primarily relying on gestures with minimal verbal input, please try to actively incorporate voice and words into your interactions.

Communication is a two-way process, and emotional exchanges such as empathy are just as important as the transfer of information. Don't focus solely on teaching specific words like "bus" or "train." Instead, try incorporating playful sounds and words that accompany actions, like "pop," "rumble," "crash," or "heave-ho." Using your voice frequently will help your child practice expressing things vocally.

Language development requires a foundation of healthy physical and mental growth. While having a cleft palate may raise additional concerns, it's important to note that, without complications, a cleft palate itself does not significantly hinder language development. Environmental factors, otitis media with effusion (OME), or speech disorders may cause slight delays in early language development, but many children catch up over a few years.

That said, various factors can affect language development, and delays might occur not only in speech but also in language comprehension. If your child has difficulties with social interaction or behavior, it's essential to address these issues appropriately. In such cases, consulting a professional institution for tailored support is highly recommended.

CHAPTER 5. CHILDCARE

CHAPTER 5. CHILDCARE

Q 82. IS IT TRUE THAT CHILDREN WITH CLEFT LIP AND PALATE EXPERIENCE SLOWER PHYSICAL GROWTH?

A There are cases where they may not gain weight adequately because they cannot consume enough milk.

Children with cleft lip and palate may experience slower physical growth, particularly in the early months of life. This is often due to feeding difficulties caused by their condition. The cleft in the lip or palate can result in weak sucking ability, making it hard for them to effectively feed. As a result, they may struggle to take in enough milk, which can lead to insufficient weight gain. In some cases, milk may even leak from the nose during feeding, further complicating the process.

To help improve feeding and encourage healthy growth, healthcare providers may offer specific recommendations. These can include using specialized bottles or nipples designed for children with cleft palate, which make it easier for them to drink. In some cases, parents may also be advised on techniques or positions that support better feeding.

Additionally, if a child has other health conditions alongside the cleft, this can also impact their overall growth and weight gain. Close monitoring and ongoing support from healthcare professionals are important to ensure that children with clefts receive the care and nutrition they need.

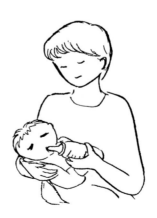

Q 83. DOES A CHILD WITH CLEFT LIP AND PALATE EXPERIENCE DELAYED SPEECH DEVELOPMENT, LEADING TO LOWER INTELLIGENCE OR SLOWER MENTAL DEVELOPMENT?

A Having cleft lip and palate alone does not necessarily result in decreased intelligence or delays in mental development. However, if there are other associated conditions in addition to the cleft lip and palate, these may include symptoms such as intellectual impairments or delays in mental development. Therefore, differences in intelligence and development will depend on the individual symptoms of each child.

How significant the differences may be is difficult to determine at birth. Over time, by observing the child's development, their condition can gradually be better understood. In fact, many individuals born with cleft lip and palate grow up without any intellectual impairments or developmental delays. There are numerous cases where individuals born with cleft lip and palate go on to lead successful lives, including taking on leadership roles in society.

In cases where there are associated conditions or symptoms that might affect intellectual or mental development, it is crucial to make an effort to minimize such impacts. This can be achieved by providing frequent verbal interaction and intellectual stimulation as early as possible. On the other hand, even without associated conditions, limited verbal interaction or inadequate intellectual stimulation can hinder the child's development. Misunderstandings about the child's abilities, such as assuming they are less capable than they are, may also negatively impact their progress.

It is recommended that families and all individuals involved in the child's upbringing remain attentive to the child's physical, mental, and intellectual development while continuing to engage with them proactively. Children often understand far more than they are able to express themselves. By offering appropriate stimulation, it is possible to support the child's steady development. Parents and caregivers are encouraged to envision the future growth of the child while cherishing each day and fostering an environment conducive to their development. This approach can help reduce delays caused by associated conditions and promote the child's overall progress.

Reference

1) Ito M. et al. Language development in children with cleft lip and palate. Part 2 Analysis using the infant mental development diagnostic method (0-2 years old). Aichi Gakuin J Dent Sci, 48(1): 21-26, 2010.

CHAPTER 5. CHILDCARE

Q 84. ARE THERE ANY RESTRICTIONS FOR CHILDREN WITH CLEFT LIP AND PALATE WHEN IT COMES TO SPORTS (E.G., ACTIVITIES THEY SHOULD AVOID)? ALSO, ARE THERE ANY AREAS THEY MIGHT STRUGGLE WITH?

A **There are no specific restrictions on sports activities solely due to cleft lip and palate. However, children with cleft lip and palate tend to frequently experience middle ear infections (commonly serous otitis media).**

For parents of children with cleft lip and palate, here's an explanation of how their condition might affect sports participation:

There are generally no specific restrictions on the types of sports children with cleft lip and palate can engage in. However, children with this condition are more prone to otitis media, particularly serous otitis media (a form of middle ear fluid buildup without pain). If your child has symptoms of ear problems, especially fluid in the ear, it is advisable to avoid swimming to prevent further complications or infections. Keep in mind that serous otitis media may not cause noticeable pain or discomfort, so regular check-ups with an otolaryngologist (ENT specialist) are essential. Children who have had ear issues in the past may experience recurrent episodes, so it's important to monitor and be cautious.

Cleft lip and palate do not inherently affect a child's athletic ability. It is a myth that children with clefts are bad at sports due to their condition. On the contrary, it is encouraged to allow children to try a variety of activities from a young age, as physical exercise is vital for their development.

From the time they start walking, children should be given opportunities to engage in physical activities like playing in parks, using playground equipment (such as slides, mats, or bars), or practicing with sports tools like rackets or balls. These activities will help them develop coordination, balance, and strength. You might discover that your child has a preference for certain activities, whether indoors or outdoors, and that's perfectly normal. The key is to support their interests and encourage exploration without hesitation.

The most important thing is to offer your child a variety of opportunities to explore physical activity, be it indoors or outside. Finding a sport, they enjoy can boost their self-confidence, which will benefit them not only in sports but also in other areas of life, including school. Encouragement, especially if they express interest in physical activity, can make a significant difference in their confidence and overall well-being.

Reference

1) Toriyama M. et al. Otolaryngology. Igaku-shoin, Tokyo, 2002.

[Q] 85. IS IT NECESSARY TO WRITE "CLEFT LIP AND PALATE" IN THE DISEASE COLUMN OF THE PRE-VACCINATION MEDICAL QUESTIONNAIRE? ARE THERE ANY PRECAUTIONS TO TAKE WHEN RECEIVING VACCINATIONS?

[A] **If "cleft lip and palate" is written in the medical history section, it can help assess the baby's overall condition, such as whether there is any regurgitation of breast milk or formula through the nose during feeding, the extent of such occurrences if present, and their impact on feeding, the respiratory system, and overall development.**
When receiving vaccinations, having a cleft lip and palate does not require special adjustments or precautions. However, providing this information may aid healthcare providers in understanding the child's health background better.

Before receiving vaccinations, it is mandatory to fill out the "pre-vaccination questionnaire" or "medical interview form" with the required details, as you likely already know. These forms ask for detailed information to comprehensively and accurately understand your child's health status. This step is essential to ensure the safe administration of vaccines.

Healthcare providers use this information to make a thorough and efficient judgment, minimizing the risk of oversight. Parents are advised to avoid omitting information or making assumptions, ensuring they fill out the form accurately and honestly.

Regarding the question, if "cleft lip and palate" is noted on the form, it provides valuable context for assessing factors like whether milk or formula regurgitates through the nose during feeding, the degree of such issues, the impact on feeding and respiratory function, and overall development. This information may also prompt careful evaluation of associated conditions, such as hearing impairment.

The pre-vaccination questionnaire is not solely for deciding whether the child can receive the vaccine. It can also serve as critical documentation to investigate the causal relationship if any adverse reactions occur post-vaccination. Vaccinations are one of many milestones in a child's growth. Observing their development holistically and providing appropriate follow-up care is vital.

Other general precautions for vaccinations include checking the child's condition and temperature on the day of the vaccination, noting recent health issues (especially within the past month), any history of seizures, allergies to medications or foods, and previous vaccinations within the last month. For more general information on vaccinations, refer to the Ministry of Health, Labor and Welfare's General Information on Vaccinations (Revised)" (2012), which is available in a Q&A format for clarity.

121

Reference
1) www.wakutin.or.jp/medical/pdf/qa2012_01.pdf

Q 86. SHOULD I CONSULT WITH KINDERGARTEN OR SCHOOL TEACHERS?

A Yes, it is recommended to inform the teachers in charge about your child's condition.

It seems that many parents do not talk to the kindergarten or school teachers about their child's condition. As a result, children may receive comments like being slow to eat during lunchtime or not reading clearly during language lessons. Some children may not mention these things at home, so parents may not be aware of them. Over time, this can lead to the child starting to dislike going to school or kindergarten. Whenever there is a change in class or grade, it is a good idea to talk to the new teacher about the child's condition.

The Japanese Cleft Palate Foundation has prepared a booklet that parents can give to teachers to help explain the condition.

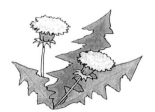

Q 87. HOW SHOULD I EXPLAIN THE POSTOPERATIVE SCAR TO MY CHILD?

A **You can explain it like this: "It's because you got hurt inside mommy's tummy, so we went to the hospital, and the doctors helped to fix it."**

In our research, we found that children start to recognize their condition as early as around age 2-3 for some, while about half of the mothers who reported having explained the condition to their child were doing so when their child was in the upper elementary grades. As a result, many children may recognize their condition but haven't received any explanation from their mothers. This can lead to situations where children don't know how to explain their condition when asked by friends about their scars at kindergarten or school, which sometimes leads to bullying.

The reason many mothers haven't explained their child's condition is often due to uncertainty about when or how to explain it, or whether they should even bring it up at all.

At our facility, we approach these situations with the following mindset. As soon as a child asks, "Why is your lip like that?" or shows concern by looking at their scar in the mirror, we recommend explaining it right away. If parents try to hide the condition, the child may pick up on it and interpret that there is something wrong or shameful about discussing it, leading them to avoid talking about it with others, which can affect their relationships with friends.

If a child asks, "Why do you have a scar?", a simple explanation like, "It's because you got hurt inside mommy's tummy, and we went to the hospital where the doctors helped to fix it," is best. This way, the child can accept the explanation and confidently share it with friends when asked, and the other children will understand as well.

The Japanese Cleft Palate Foundation has published a picture book, "Chi-chan's Mouth" (written by Mami Watanabe), to help explain the condition to children.

123

CHAPTER 5. CHILDCARE

Q 88. HOW SHOULD I EXPLAIN TO MY CHILD'S FRIENDS?

A It would be helpful to explain that they might have similar scars in the future, so it's not something special.

If a child asks a question, for example, "Why does ○○-chan speak strangely?" you could say, "Right now, ○○-chan has an illness and are undergoing training. It might seem a bit odd, but being treated, and will get better soon, so let's help ○○-chan until then." Or, "It's a speech condition, and it's being treated, so ○○-chan get better in time."

"You never know when someone might develop a speech disorder and lose the ability to speak. ○○-chan is doing much better now than before. Since they're working hard now, I think ○○-chan will be even better next year"

If a child asks, "Why is there a scar above the mouth?" parents should respond calmly and naturally, "That's because you had an injury when you were in your mother's belly, and the doctors at the university hospital treated it, leaving a scar. ○○-chan didn't cry at all during that time, so you were really brave." You could also say, "The face isn't like clothes, so people often get facial injuries in traffic accidents or sports. Everyone, be careful!"

By explaining this way, children can understand that they might also have similar scars and that it's not something special.

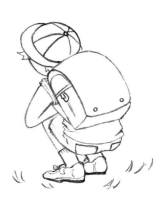

124

Q 89. "I WOULD LIKE TO HEAR ABOUT THE EXPERIENCE OF RAISING A CHILD WITH THE SAME CONDITION..."

A There are 'parent associations' and 'patient associations' in various regions.

There are parent and patient associations for cleft lip and palate patients across Japan, engaging in various activities. By joining a parent association, you can hear about various experiences. For inquiries about local parent associations and patient associations, please contact the Japanese Cleft Palate Foundation (NPO).

There are also many organizations abroad, and the International Cleft Lip and Palate Association introduces such organizations. However, in this case, communication will be conducted in English."

Q 90. "I WOULD LIKE TO CORRESPOND WITH MOTHERS OF CHILDREN WITH CLEFT LIP AND PALATE ABROAD..."

A Recently, various parent associations and support groups seem to have started pages on social networks.

As a parent of a child with a cleft lip and palate, you may find it helpful to connect with other parents who are going through similar experiences. Recently, many parent associations and support groups have started using social media to create spaces where families can share advice, stories, and support.

For example, the International Cleft Lip and Palate Foundation (ICPF) has a social networking platform specifically for parents of children with cleft lip and palate. These online groups are great places to exchange tips on managing cleft conditions, share your personal experiences, and learn from others around the world. Topics might include how to manage feeding challenges, prepare for surgeries, or deal with emotional and social concerns.

Additionally, we have created a page for parents of children with cleft lip and palate on Facebook. This page serves as another way for families to connect, support each other, and share valuable resources. Joining these groups can be a great way to feel less alone in your journey, gain useful information, and find emotional support from people who truly understand. (https://www.facebook.com/pages/International-Cleft-Lip-and-Palate-Foundation-ICPF/587964304581148?fref=ts)

CHAPTER 5. CHILDCARE

Q 91. ARE THERE ANY CLEFT LIP AN PALATE NGO'S OVERSEAS?

A There are many organizations around the world.

In the United States, there is a program called "Operation Smile" that provides support to children with clefts. The parent group called "Smile," which, while not specialized in cleft lip and palate, offers support for all types of clefts, whether congenital or acquired.

In Canada, there is an organization called "About Face," run by children with facial differences, their parents, and families.

Another organization, the "22q Foundation", supports individuals with 22q11.2 deletion syndrome and is operated by parents, individuals with the condition, and professionals.

These organizations operate worldwide. Since "Operation Smile" is active in the United States, they have connections with parent groups across many countries. If you are seeking a parent group in a specific country, you can reach out to these organizations.

Q 92. DO CHILDREN WITH CLEFT LIP AND PALATE PASS GAS A LOT?

A It is not common, but it can occur when air is sucked in together with the milk at the cleft area and swallowed during breastfeeding.

Having a cleft lip or palate does not directly cause excessive gas or bloating. However, it can happen if air is sucked in with the milk during breastfeeding, leading to the baby swallowing both air and milk. In most cases, this is not a major concern, but improper breastfeeding techniques can sometimes cause issues.

It is important to check the breastfeeding position. Make sure to prop the baby up slightly and allow breaks for burping during feeding. If these steps are not followed properly, it may lead to increased gas, insufficient milk intake, or in some cases, vomiting (spitting up).

Q 93. IS THERE A MOVIE TO HELP UNDERSTAND CLEFT LIP AND PALATE?

A There is "Kazuko's Departure" (Eizousha).

For parents of children with cleft lip and palate, the film "*Kazuko's Departure*" (Eizousha) can be a helpful resource. Produced by the "Tanpopo-kai" cleft lip and palate support group, this 60-minute film focuses on the story of a young girl named Kazuko who lives with a cleft lip and palate. The film is designed to provide insight into the challenges and experiences associated with this condition, offering a perspective that can help families better understand the emotional and physical aspects of having a child with a cleft.

The film is available for rental for a fee and also comes in video format. Additionally, a DVD version has been created to support informed consent, particularly for parents who have been given a prenatal diagnosis of cleft lip and palate. This resource is particularly useful for those seeking more information and understanding prior to making medical decisions.

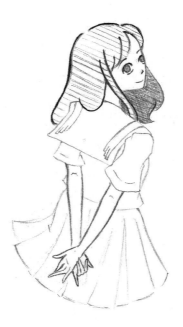

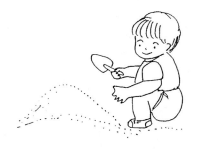

CHAPTER *6.* *TREATMENT COST, SOCIAL SERVICES*

CHAPTER 6. TREATMENT COST, SOCIAL SERVICES

Q 94. PLEASE TELL ME ABOUT THE INSURANCE SYSTEMS AVAILABLE FOR PATIENTS WITH CLEFT LIP AND PALATE

A **There are two types of systems: Medical Aid for Development and Medical Aid for Rehabilitation.**

For patients under a certain age, Medical Aid for Development applies to those with cleft lip and palate who have significant occlusion disorders or related issues. For patients above a certain age, Medical Aid for Rehabilitation is available.

However, it does not apply to all individuals with cleft lip and palate. After surgery for cleft lip and palate, it is applicable only in cases where speech disorders or significant malocclusion are observed."

Q 95. WHAT PROCEDURES SHOULD BE APPLIED FOR AFTER THE BIRTH OF A CHILD WITH A CLEFT LIP AND PALATE?

A **Please consult your attending physician.**

Outpatient treatments such as feeding Hotz plates or palatal expanders can be applied for, depending on the circumstances. The specific period varies by municipality from 6 months to 1 year. For those undergoing treatment using oral appliances like feeding plates or expanders, it is possible to apply.

For patients planning to undergo their first cleft lip surgery, applications should be submitted promptly after a hospital admission date is determined. Please note that a new application may be required before subsequent hospitalizations. The eligibility period for Medical Aid for Development depends on the municipality and typically ranges from several months to a few years after the impression-taking date.

If hospitalization is canceled or surgery is postponed due to unavoidable circumstances after completing the procedures, please consult regarding the necessary steps under the self-reliance medical system. It is not automatically applied. Please reapply before being readmitted to the hospital.

For patients receiving treatment in the orthodontics department, a reapplication is required, so please ensure to submit the necessary documents.

Rehabilitation medical aid is only applicable in cases where a significant chewing disability is diagnosed post-surgery. It does not apply to all patients with cleft lip and palate. Please consult your attending physician for more details. Applications are valid for a period of one year from the date of approval. If continued treatment is needed, reapplication will be necessary.

Q 96. CAN YOU TELL ME ABOUT MEDICAL AID FOR SELF-RELIANCE? DOES IT MAKE MEDICAL EXPENSES FREE IF APPLIED?
ALSO, UNTIL WHAT AGE IS IT APPLICABLE?

A **For detailed information, please contact your local health center.**

When children under age of 18th receive treatment at facilities designated as developmental medical institutions by the Ministry of Health, Labor and Welfare, part or all of the patient's medical expenses may be subsidized.

However, depending on the amount of income tax paid, patients may be required to cover part or all of the medical expenses themselves.

For more details, please contact your local public health center.

Q 97. WHAT IS THE COST OF THE FIRST AND CORRECTIVE SURGERIES?
ALSO, ARE THE MEDICAL AID FOR SELF-RELIANCE OR HEALTH INSURANCE SYSTEMS APPLICABLE?

A **Please contact your nearest municipal office for more information.**

Health insurance is applicable. If the institution is designated, programs such as infant medical care and developmental medical care can be used, and surgeries are generally free of charge. However, if the guardian's income is high or if a private room is requested during hospitalization, there may be additional costs for the difference in bed fees.

Please contact your nearest municipal office for more information.

131

CHAPTER 6. TREATMENT COST, SOCIAL SERVICES

Q 98. FOR INDIVIDUALS AGED 18 AND OLDER, WHAT IS THE COST OF SECONDARY SURGERIES?

A Since it is outside the scope of medical aid for development, except in special cases, there will be a need for partial payment of treatment costs. Additionally, the costs may vary depending on the insurance plan and the type of surgery, so please contact the facility for more details.

For individuals aged 18 and older, medical aid for development is no longer applicable. Except in special cases, partial payment of treatment costs will be required.

For example, the approximate cost for cleft lip and nose correction surgery at our facility is as follows (as of October 2014): Insurance points 45,000 -65,000. In the case of 10% of copayment,

- 10% share: ¥53,000 to ¥72,800
- 20% share: ¥97,800 to ¥137,800
- 30% share: ¥142,800 to ¥202,800

This does not include the cost for a private room or separate room if requested. Additionally, if a cosmetic surgery or self-funded surgery is performed at a cosmetic surgery clinic, the costs may vary significantly depending on the individual hospital.

The amount of payment required depends on the insurance plan and the specifics of the surgery, including the type of surgery, hospital stay, tests, and medications.

Please note that this is only an estimate and the final amount may differ.

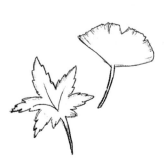

[Q] 99. WHAT IS THE COST OF ORTHODONTIC TREATMENT, PROSTHETIC DENTAL TREATMENT, AND IMPLANT TREATMENT? ALSO, ARE MEDICAL AID FOR SELF-RELIANCE AND HEALTH INSURANCE SYSTEMS APPLICABLE?

[A] **For prosthetic treatment of missing teeth after orthodontic treatment, there may be cases where treatment can or cannot be covered by insurance. To apply for the self-reliance medical system, a diagnosis by a medical professional is required. Please confirm this with your attending physician or your local public health center or municipal office.**

For the treatment of cleft lip and palate patients, insurance treatment is generally applied. Even for orthodontic treatment, which is usually not covered by insurance, health insurance is recognized for cleft lip and palate treatment.

In recent years, there are systems like Children's Medical Care and Infant Medical Care to assist with medical expenses for children. These systems help cover the out-of-pocket expenses for insurance-covered treatment, with local governments shouldering the costs. However, this system varies by municipality in terms of eligible age and the application process, so it is necessary to confirm with the local government (some municipalities have expanded the eligible age for inpatient treatment costs).

Therefore, depending on the municipality, the situation may differ, but there is public financial assistance for medical expenses up to a certain age, significantly reducing the economic burden on patients and their guardians.

Additionally, there is the Self-reliance Medical Aid System supported by the government. This system is a public cost-sharing program that helps reduce the out-of-pocket expenses for medical treatments aimed at alleviating or removing physical and mental disabilities, including those for cleft lip and palate patients.

Regarding treatments for cleft lip and palate, Medical Aid for Development is applicable for children with physical disabilities, including surgeries to remove or alleviate those disabilities under the age of 18.

This is not a completely cost-free system, and the cost-sharing for the user depends on the materials used and the treatment method, similar to prosthetic treatments. The use of precious metals or porcelain (ceramics) can affect the cost. However, there are facility standards for this application, and it is not available at all dental care facilities.

For treatments that can certainly be expected to have an effect, the user's burden will be determined

133

CHAPTER 6. TREATMENT COST, SOCIAL SERVICES

based on income, but if the income is too high, insurance coverage may not apply. Additionally, for cases involving implant treatments, similar constraints apply, and these treatments may not be readily covered by insurance.

For patients with cleft lip and palate, to apply for medical aid, a diagnosis by a medical professional is required, and the treatment must meet specific conditions such as physical disabilities under the Disability Welfare Act.

In terms of implant treatments, the current situation is that insurance coverage is less likely to be applied, especially in cases of cleft lip and palate. However, there have been efforts for expansion in coverage for treatments like speech and language function disorders associated with cleft lip and palate, including necessary orthodontic treatments since 2012. This includes possible coverage for bone defects caused by tumors, injuries, or congenital anomalies.

However, this system is not applicable at all dental medical institutions due to facility standards, and there is also a restriction that the patient must be missing more than one-third of the jaw. Therefore, it is difficult to apply to patients with only one or two missing teeth, as is often the case with cleft lip and palate patients. It is necessary to confirm the eligibility and application process with your local health center or municipal office for further details.

Efforts are ongoing to improve access to these treatments across healthcare professionals and administrators.

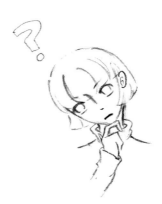

[Q] 100. WHAT IS THE COST OF SPEECH THERAPY? ALSO, ARE MEDICAL AID FOR SELF-RELIANCE AND HEALTH INSURANCE SYSTEMS APPLICABLE?

[A] **If the hospital provides treatment by a speech-language pathologist, health insurance is applicable. Please confirm with the hospital first.**

If the hospital provides treatment by a speech-language pathologist, health insurance is applicable. Please confirm with the hospital first. Speech therapy is calculated on an hourly basis. Depending on the size, you will be required to pay approximately ¥2,000 to ¥3,000 per session."

The main target of speech therapy is infants and young children, and it is a condition that the child must undergo treatment for certain disabilities that could remain in the future. The procedures are handled by the relevant departments in each municipality.

There is a Child Medical Expense Assistance System in each municipality. This system subsidizes the out-of-pocket medical expenses for your child. To use this system, your child must first be enrolled in health insurance.

The target age and details of the assistance vary depending on the municipality, so please check with your local municipality's office for the procedures.

Self-reliance medical aid is a system that subsidizes part of the costs for medical treatments that improve symptoms in children with physical disabilities or diseases. In the case of cleft lip and palate, it applies to inpatient treatments like surgical procedures and orthodontic treatment, but it does not apply to speech therapy.

In the case of speech therapy, the costs are fully out-of-pocket. The costs vary depending on the facility, so please confirm with each facility.

135

CHAPTER 6. TREATMENT COST, SOCIAL SERVICES

[Q] 101. CAN A DISABILITY CERTIFICATE BE RECEIVED IN THE CASE OF CLEFT LIP AND PALATE?

[A] **It can be obtained if there is recognition of a disability in speech/ language function or masticatory function.**

A disability certificate is issued if one of the following 12 types of disabilities is recognized, and the degree of disability determines the classification:

The types of disabilities include: visual impairment, hearing impairment, speech/language function impairment, mastication function impairment, physical disability, internal disabilities such as heart function impairment, respiratory function impairment, intestinal function impairment, small intestine function impairment, immune function impairment, and liver function impairment.

In the case of cleft lip and palate, recognition of speech/language function impairment or mastication function impairment may apply. These diagnoses require examination by a speech-language pathologist or doctor, so please consult with your attending physician.

[Q] 102. DOES OBTAINING A DISABILITY CERTIFICATE DISADVANTAGE YOU WHEN SEEKING EMPLOYMENT?

[A] **Obtaining a disability certificate does not necessarily disadvantage you when seeking employment.**

The Ministry of Health, Labor, and Welfare has a policy for promoting the employment of people with disabilities, called the "Disabled Employment Promotion Act." This requires companies to hire people with disabilities, amounting to 2.0% of their total workforce (disability employment rate system). Therefore, when seeking employment, you may be able to secure a position within this employment quota. It does not necessarily put you at a disadvantage.

Q 103. WHAT IS A REHABILITATION HANDICAPPED PERSON'S HANDBOOK?

A **Since the Welfare Law for Persons with Intellectual Disabilities does not specifically mention an intellectual disability handbook, each local government has its own criteria for assessment and certification.**

The so-called physical disability handbook is outlined in the Disability Welfare Law, but there are some issues arising from the differing assessments and certifications made by each local government.

For individuals under a certain age, they are assessed by a child consultation center, particularly in cities like Nagoya, where it is referred to as the "Welfare Protection Handicapped Person's Handbook." For individuals 18 years and older, the intellectual disability certification is done by an intellectual disability welfare organization.

The classifications of the disability and severity vary, with some individuals being granted the certification based on different assessments for mild, moderate, or severe conditions.

Reference

1) Wellnet Nagoya (Disability Welfare Handbook)

http://www.kaigo-wel.city.nagoya.jp/view/wel/leaflet/f19a_02

Q 104. WHY DO MEDICAL COST SUBSIDIES DIFFER BETWEEN MUNICIPALITIES?

A **The eligibility for application, as well as the application forms and methods, vary by municipality. Please contact your local health department or similar office for more information.**

Some municipalities have their own medical subsidy programs (for example, infant medical cost assistance, specific disease medical cost assistance, infertility treatment assistance, developmental medical cost assistance, medical cost assistance for persons with disabilities, and medical cost assistance for single-parent households).

Depending on your child's condition and family circumstances, eligibility for application, as well as the required application forms and methods, may vary by municipality. Please be sure to contact your local health department or similar office for details.

CHAPTER 6. TREATMENT COST, SOCIAL SERVICES

[Q] 105. PLEASE TELL ME ABOUT THE EDUCATIONAL INSURANCE THAT CHILDREN WITH CLEFT LIP AND PALATE CAN GET

[A] **For more information, please contact the Japanese Cleft Palate Foundation's telephone support.**

Although there are few insurance companies that sell education insurance, you can enroll in education insurance that you can take out for the purpose of saving for education. However, it is thought that you cannot enroll in the medical insurance that comes with it if you have a cleft lip and palate.

For more information, please contact the Japanese Cleft Palate Foundation's telephone support (052-757-4312). Inquiries are accepted free of charge.

[Q] 106. PLEASE TELL ME ABOUT LIFE INSURANCE THAT CHILDREN WITH CLEFT LIP AND PALATE CAN ENROLL IN

[A] **You can inquire with individual insurance companies or for more details, please contact the Japanese Cleft Palate Foundation's phone support.**

Life insurance with the child as the insured may not be available if the child has conditions such as cleft lip and palate or heart complications, or if there is a planned surgery. However, some insurance companies may allow enrollment without conditions. You can inquire with individual insurance companies or for more details, please contact the Japanese Cleft Palate Foundation's phone support at (052-757-4312). Inquiries are accepted for free.

Q 107. EVEN WITH A CONGENITAL DISEASE, IS IT POSSIBLE TO JOIN MEDICAL INSURANCE IN THE FUTURE?

A For more details, please contact the Japanese Cleft Palate Foundation's phone support.

Not many insurance companies allow enrollment. However, there are insurance companies you can enroll but pre-existing conditions, including those currently being treated (such as lip/palate, teeth, tongue, and submandibular glands), may not be covered. Some insurance companies exclude coverage for the specific diseases.

For more details, please contact the Japanese Cleft Palate Foundation's phone support (052-757-4312). Inquiries are free of charge.

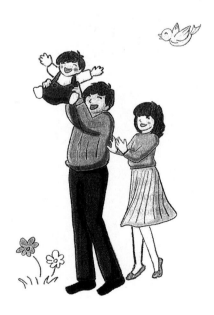

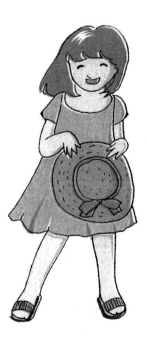

CHAPTER 7. FEEDING PROBLEMS

CHAPTER 7. FEEDING PROBLEMS

108. PLEASE TELL ME ABOUT FEEDING CHILDREN WITH CLEFT LIP AND PALATE

A Please refer to the following.

Can babies with cleft lip and palate drink milk or breastfeed normally? Please tell me about baby bottles and breast pumps.

For babies with cleft lip and palate, special bottles and nipples are recommended to support feeding. One example is the Pigeon feeding bottle for cleft lip and palate babies (**Fig. 1**). This bottle is equipped with an anti-reflux valve, enabling feeding even if the baby lacks suction power, as the milk flows with gentle chewing.

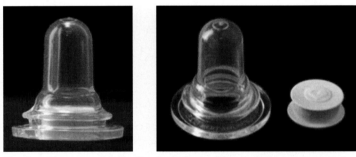

Fig.1 Pigeon nipple for babies with cleft lip and palate

For babies with cleft palate, due to air leakage from the nose, suction is often challenging. The specialized nipples in these bottles are designed to make feeding easier, with a larger size for better sealing and a silicone nipple with varying thickness (thicker on the nasal side and thinner on the tongue side) to optimize milk flow.

Other options include the Medela Special Needs Feeder (**Fig. 2**), Chuchu bottles (**Fig. 3**), or Bean Stalk Nipples (**Fig. 4**), all designed for babies struggling with regular feeding. If the baby has neurological or jaw-related issues, oral feeding might remain difficult even with these tools. In such cases, consult your healthcare provider for guidance.

For additional support, refer to specialized feeding bottles and nipples available for cleft lip and

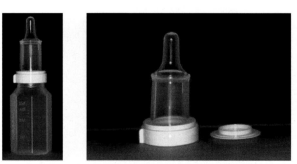

Fig. 2 Medela Special Needs Feeder

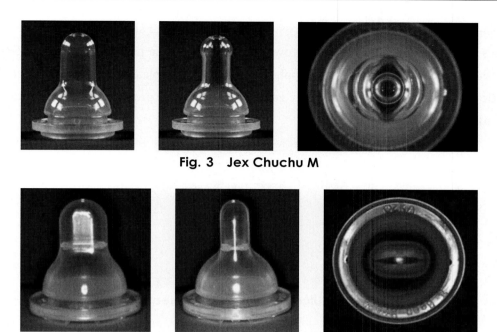

Fig. 3   Jex Chuchu M

Fig. 4   Otsuka Pharmaceutical Bean Stalk Nipples

palate patients.

Regarding breast pumps: The presence of a cleft lip and/or palate in your child does not affect the choice of a breast pump. You can use any commercially available pump that you find convenient and comfortable.

How to calculate feeding volume and milk requirements

The daily milk requirement is approximately 100 mL per kilogram of body weight. If this amount is not met, supplementary hydration via feeding tubes or intravenous fluids may be necessary. For healthy growth, the recommended milk intake ranges from 150 to 200 mL per kilogram of body weight.

The amount of milk per feeding session can be calculated by dividing the total daily requirement by the number of feedings. For example, if your baby feeds 8 times a day, divide the daily requirement by 8 to determine the amount per session.

The feeding time per session should ideally be around 15-20 minutes. Prolonging feeding sessions beyond this can lead to fatigue and may not increase intake due to the baby feeling full from earlier feeding.

What is a Hotz plate?

A Hotz plate (palatal plate) is an orthodontic appliance designed primarily for infants with cleft palates. Since a cleft palate causes air leakage between the nose and mouth, it becomes difficult for the baby to suck milk effectively. Additionally, the nipple may press against the nasal septum, potentially causing ulcers (**Fig. 5**). Specialized nipples can also help by preventing the tip from entering the nasal cavity and protecting the nasal septum from ulcers. The Hotz plate serves not only to address these issues but also to correct alveolar discrepancies.

143

The plate is typically worn from an early stage until palate repair surgery is performed. However, it requires fine adjustments as the child grows and for orthodontic purposes, so regular follow-ups with the doctor are crucial. Dentures or appliances like the Hotz plate are designed to guide growth in specific directions by creating necessary gaps, but they may be prone to becoming dislodged due to these adjustments.

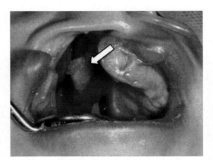

Fig. 5   Ulceration of the nasal septum

The Hotz plate (**Fig. 6**) covers the cleft palate, reducing air leakage and protecting the nasal septum. It facilitates feeding and can improve the baby's breathing during feeding.

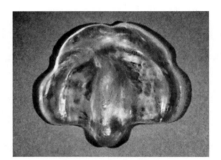

Fig. 6   Hotz plate

In cases where the baby cannot feed effectively, tube feeding (nutritional intake through a nasal tube) may be required. Feeding methods depend on the baby's condition and overall health, so it is important to consult with your doctor to determine the most suitable approach.

The name Hotz plate is derived from its developer, Margaret Hotz.

I am currently giving my baby milk through a tube in his nose. Will he be able to drink from his mouth in the future?

It is important to prevent the child from losing their natural sucking reflex. However, in cases where there are issues with the cranial nervous system or micrognathia, feeding movements may not function as effectively.

When tube feeding through the nose is used, oral intake may become possible as the child grows, especially if the jaw develops to a sufficient size. The timing of this depends on the child's age, but efforts should focus on enhancing suction strength (the ability to suck).

For children with a cleft palate, insufficient suction strength due to the cleft can be addressed by starting with thickened baby food and gradually transitioning to liquids after weaning. Prematurely forcing oral feeding is not recommended.

If the only issue is insufficient suction strength, switching nipples or using a Hotz plate may allow the child to feed orally. Prolonged tube feeding can inhibit the development of natural feeding movements, so transitioning away from tube feeding as early as possible is desirable.

If there are no other issues, encourage oral feeding as much as possible, and supplement with tube feeding for any remaining milk. Advancing oral intake helps minimize the risk of aspiration or choking. It is crucial to consult with your doctor rather than making independent judgments and to start training under professional guidance.

Even if oral intake has not progressed, encourage feeding movements by giving the child an empty nipple or pacifier while administering milk through the tube. This helps prevent the child from losing their natural sucking reflex.

What should I do if the child refuses to drink milk but consumes vegetable juice or other beverages?

If the child can drink vegetable juice or other liquids, it indicates that their feeding function remains intact. Start with diluted beverages and gradually transition to milk, using the methods described earlier.

In cases where the child skips feedings and refuses to drink, try diluting vegetable juice or similar liquids, and slowly transition them to plain boiled water. Once they are accustomed to plain water, introduce thin milk and gradually increase its concentration. This approach can be effective.

For children who have developed taste preferences from exposure to various flavors, it's recommended to return to just milk and plain boiled water (sayu). When they become hungry or thirsty, they may naturally begin drinking milk or boiled water again.

If the child can consume other liquids, it suggests that feeding movements are still possible. Early intervention is key to achieving success.

How do I burp a child with cleft lip and/or palate?

Burping can be done in the same way as usual, even for children with cleft lip and/or palate. However, if milk comes out during burping, it may also come out from the nose. After burping, gently clean the mouth and nose to maintain hygiene.

CHAPTER 7. FEEDING PROBLEMS

Q 109. WHEN SHOULD WE START INTRODUCING SOLID FOODS, AND HOW SHOULD WE PROCEED?

A There are individual differences in a baby's development, but the following guidelines can be used as a reference.

Babies' development varies from child to child, but around 5 to 6 months of age, you may notice the following signs:

1. Neck stability
2. Showing interest in food
3. Ability to sit up with support
4. Putting objects, like a spoon, into their mouth

Once you observe that your baby is pushing less food out with their tongue, it's a good time to start introducing solid foods.

Around 5-6 months (early weaning period)

- Frequency: Once a day
- Food form: Mashed (yogurt-like) consistency
- Start with one scoop at a time and gradually increase the amount as your baby gets used to it.

During this time, the goal is not to focus on quantity but to introduce new flavors other than milk.

The purpose is to help your baby learn to close their lips and swallow baby food. Gently touch your baby's lower lip with the spoon to encourage them to close their upper lip and scoop the food up.

After starting weaning, continue to offer your baby as much breast milk or formula as they want during the early and middle stages of weaning.

Around 7-8 months (mid-weaning period)

- Frequency: Twice a day
- Food form: Soft enough to be crushed with the tongue (similar in texture to tofu)

During this stage, babies can begin eating small, soft pieces of food that can be mashed up.

This is the stage when you can introduce more ingredients, such as chicken and lean fish. It's also a good time to start paying closer attention to nutritional balance.

Around 9-11 months (late weaning)

- Frequency: 3 times a day
- Food form: Soft enough to be crushed with gums (approximately the size of a banana)

At this stage, the baby's tongue can move from side to side, in addition to moving back and forth

146

and up and down. Once the side-to-side motion is developed, the baby will be able to crush food with their gums and eat it. Be cautious with food textures; if the food is not suitable, it may be swallowed whole.

Around 12-18 months

- Frequency: 3 times a day
- Food type: Soft enough to be chewed with gums (similar to the hardness of a meatball)

At this stage, let your baby enjoy the experience of eating with their hands, such as by offering rice balls. A good indicator that weaning is complete is when your baby can bite food with their gums and get most of their nutrients from meals. Once your baby turns one year old, it's fine to introduce milk. However, it should be given in a cup, not a bottle, with a recommended intake of 300-400 ml per day. If your baby dislikes milk, there's no need to force them to drink it. Gradually introduce it through dishes like boiled milk or potato salad to help them get used to it.

Basically, the approach should be the same as for healthy children

While some may worry that special ingredients or food patterns are necessary, the weaning process should generally follow the same steps as for healthy children. However, some children with cleft palates may experience difficulty during the middle stage of weaning. It may take some time, but feeding food according to the baby's age is important. Additionally, food may sometimes pass through the roof of the child's mouth and into the nose, causing it to leak out. In such cases, adding a little potato starch or a thickening agent can help reduce the amount of food that enters the nose.

CHAPTER 7. FEEDING PROBLEMS

[Q] 110. PLEASE TELL ME ABOUT THE DIET (EATING HABITS) AFTER SURGERY FOR CLEFT LIP AND CLEFT PALATE. ALSO, WILL THE BABY BE ABLE TO BREASTFEED IMMEDIATELY AFTER THE SURGERY?

[A] **Depending on the healing condition of the surgical site, a soft diet is recommended for about a month post-surgery. Whether the baby can breastfeed or not, a bottle should have been used before the surgery to ensure that the baby can take breast milk or formula as needed.**

If a child is able to breastfeed before the surgery, they may be able to continue breastfeeding after the cleft lip surgery. However, especially immediately after the surgery, there is a possibility of causing slight misalignment of the sutures, which can affect healing.

Post-surgery, the sutures may be removed in about 7 to 10 days. After a cleft palate surgery, while it is possible to breastfeed, there may be pain, and the stitches on the lip may still be tender. Direct contact of the lips with the wound site could irritate the healing area, so caution is needed.

Whether the baby is able to breastfeed or not, a bottle should have been used before surgery to adjust the intake of breast milk or formula. Depending on the timing of the surgery, it may also mark the start of weaning, and transitioning to solid foods usually follows.

If the baby is unable to take any food, intravenous fluids may be necessary to prevent dehydration following surgery.

In case, if the amount of food does not increase significantly, tube feeding (inserting a tube from the nose to the stomach to provide liquid food) may be used in conjunction.

Around 3 days post-surgery, as the swelling and redness of the surgical site begin to subside, the amount of food gradually increases. To reduce physical stimulation to the wound, soft food textures are introduced first. A splint is placed on the hard palate to protect the surgical site and minimize food contact with the wound. Depending on the healing progress of the wound, soft food textures are generally recommended for about 1 month after surgery.

Q 111. CAN A 9-MONTH-OLD CHILD WITH A CLEFT PALATE DRINK FROM A STRAW?

A After the cleft palate surgery, once the cleft is closed, it becomes possible for the child to practice sucking with a straw as part of functional recovery.

To use a straw, it is important to support the straw with the lips and keep the gap between the straw and the lips closed. Coordination of the lips, tongue, cheeks, and soft palate is required to create negative pressure in the oral cavity, which is essential for sucking liquids from the straw.

Once this is achieved, the child can start drinking liquids from the straw. However, children with a cleft palate may have difficulty forming negative pressure in the oral cavity due to the cleft in the soft and hard palate, making sucking difficult. In such cases, support such as squeezing a straw pack to assist with drinking may help.

If the cleft is large, it may be difficult to create negative pressure in the oral cavity, but with practice, it may become possible around 18 months to 2 years of age when cleft palate surgery is performed. It is important to note that sucking is not achieved through surgery alone; it requires practice using the straw to regain function.

This practice typically begins around 6 months of age when weaning foods are introduced. Using a flexible straw can make it easier for the lips to support the straw, especially if the cleft is small. Palate repair surgery helps to close the cleft and improve the ability to suck.

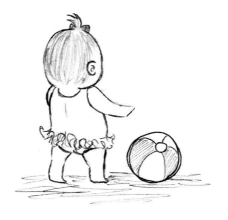

CHAPTER 7. FEEDING PROBLEMS

[Q] 112. EVEN AFTER UNDERGOING CLEFT PALATE SURGERY, FOOD IS LEAKING FROM MY CHILD'S NOSE...

[A] **If the palate (the upper part of the mouth) is completely closed, this issue will gradually improve, so there is no need to worry. If there is a hole in the palate, it is better to wait until the child has grown somewhat before performing a closure surgery.**

When cleft palate (upper part of the mouth) has been completely closed by surgery

However, if the soft palate's movement is good but the nasal cavity closure function (the ability to close the space between the mouth and nose) is still insufficient after surgery, food may leak into the nose during feeding. This occurs because the nasal cavity cannot be effectively closed. In most cases, this issue will gradually improve as the muscles of the soft palate become stronger, so there is no need to worry.

If there is a hole (fistula) in the palate

The main purpose of cleft palate surgery is to achieve nasal cavity closure function. This involves a surgery that moves most of the mucous membrane and muscles of the palate towards the back. In cases of a large cleft, a hole may form in the front due to insufficient tissue. Also, if the surgery was done considering upper jaw development using a specific technique, a hole (fistula) may remain at the front. This can lead to food leakage through the nose and unpleasant odors from food residues. This hole, which is usually quite large, can be closed, so there is no need to worry. However, even if the closure is performed early, if orthodontic treatment later widens the dental arch, a hole may reappear. If nasal leakage or speech problems persist, it is recommended to first use a closure appliance and then consider closure surgery once the child has grown enough.

150

Q 113. WHAT IS ESOPHAGEAL REFLUX DISEASE?

A It refers to the condition where stomach contents flow back into the esophagus, leading to various symptoms (complications).

In newborns, gastroesophageal reflux (GER) refers to the condition where milk is expelled during burping immediately after feeding. It is important to try methods such as keeping the baby upright and encouraging burping.

For infants with cleft lip and palate, only regurgitation and spillage of milk from the mouth may be observed without any respiratory symptoms. This happens due to the immature closure of the lower esophageal sphincter, leading to frequent burping as they often swallow air along with milk.

As for complications, digestive symptoms like vomiting, diarrhea, poor feeding, and respiratory symptoms like chronic coughing, wheezing, and repeated respiratory infections may occur. For these infants, excessive testing is generally not necessary. Instead, observation with family understanding is important. However, if vomiting continues after 2 year of age, further examination is needed to check for possible underlying issues.

It is a physiological condition that typically improves by around 3 months of age. If vomiting persists or respiratory symptoms arise, it is essential to confirm the diagnosis with a specialist.

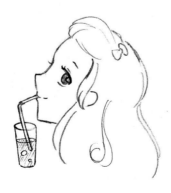

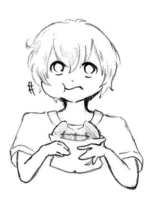

CHAPTER *8.* *EAR PROBLEMS*

CHAPTER 8. EAR PROBLEMS

Q 114. WHEN SHOULD WE START VISITING AN ENT (EAR, NOSE, AND THROAT) SPECIALIST?

A It is sufficient to start around 6 months of age, but it is recommended to visit an ENT specialist at least once before the child turns 1 year old.

For children with cleft lip and palate, the first visit to the ENT (Ear, Nose, and Throat) specialist is typically recommended when the neck stabilizes (around 2-6 months). Before the neck stabilizes, it may be challenging to assess due to instability in the head and neck. However, if there is wheezing or signs of breathing difficulties, such as inspiratory wheezing, it may indicate laryngospasm (**Fig.1, 2**), or other congenital conditions such as glottic stenosis (**Fig. 3**) or tracheal stenosis, and an early visit to either a pediatrician or ENT specialist is recommended.

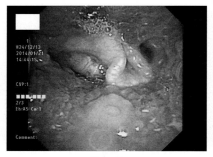

Fig. 1   Fig. 2

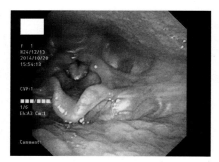

Fig. 3

In cases of cleft lip and palate, the risk of middle ear effusion (fluid in the ear) increases around 6-9 months of age, so an ENT check-up at least once is advised by 1 year of age.

If a newborn hearing screening results in a "needs re-examination" recommendation, it's important to visit an ENT specialist who can conduct more detailed hearing tests as soon as possible.

This approach ensures early diagnosis and appropriate management of potential hearing or breathing issues related to cleft lip and palate.

Q 115. IS THERE ANYTHING TO BE AWARE OF FROM AN ENT PERSPECTIVE BEFORE THE SURGERY?

A Before the lip repair surgery, it is recommended to apply "surgical tape" or "band-aids" to the cleft lip area.

If cleft lip occurs alone without cleft palate, the impact on breastfeeding is minimal. However, for children with a large cleft lip or bilateral cleft lip, it is more difficult to close the lip, which can lead to difficulty in breastfeeding. Therefore, before the cleft lip surgery, it is recommended to apply "surgical tape" or "band-aids" to the cleft lip area. (**Fig. 1**) Tape can cause a rash or promote infection, thus it is important to always keep the area clean.

In the case of a child with a cleft lip and cleft palate, there is a concern about the function of the Eustachian tube, which may be affected by abnormalities (60%) in the movement of the soft palate and the muscles associated with it.

As previously mentioned, during the first 6 months after birth, there is an increased risk of developing otitis media with effusion due to the opening of the Eustachian tube, so it is recommended that you visit an otolaryngologist between 6 and 9 months of age, or at least by 1 year of age to check the presence of absence serous otitis media.

Additionally, when a cold syndrome or acute rhinitis occurs, symptoms such as watery nasal discharge or purulent discharge may appear. If nasal discharge is observed, early consultation with an ENT specialist is recommended for nasal care and to maintain cleanliness of the nasal cavity and nasopharynx. If a child has a lot of nasal discharge, persistent nasal treatment at an otolaryngologist will help prevent serous otitis media.

Reference
1) Inuzuka E., Yoshioka T., Horibe S., Naito T. Statistical observation of serous otitis media during primary cleft palate surgery. Practica Oto-Rhino-Laryngologica, 106 (10): 833-891, 2013.

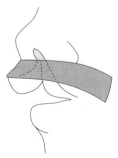

Fig. 1 Tape pasted on lips

Q 116. PLEASE TELL ME ABOUT OTITIS MEDIA WITH EFFUSION

A The details are provided below.

Why are children with cleft palates more prone to otitis media with effusion?

Children with cleft palates often have abnormal muscle function of the palatal muscles, such as the palatopharyngeus and levator veli palatini muscles, as well as an open Eustachian tube. This leads to difficulties in closing the Eustachian tube properly, and as a result, they are prone to the development of otitis media with effusion (OME). Moreover, the Eustachian tube often remains in a relatively open state in these children, which is a major contributing factor. Without proper closure and ventilation, the middle ear is at greater risk of developing fluid buildup, leading to otitis media with effusion. Thus, due to the dysfunction of the Eustachian tube, which fails to regulate the pressure within the middle ear cavity effectively. The middle ear cavity tends to develop negative pressure, making it more susceptible to the accumulation of fluid (effusion). As the fluid builds up, it may result in otitis media with effusion. (**Fig. 1**)

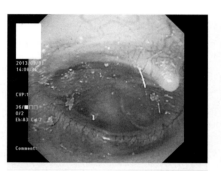
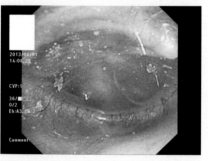
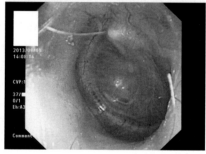

Fig. 1 The line between air and fluid in the middle ear, which looks like a thin, hairline gap

Is a child most susceptible to otitis media with effusion?

In our experiences, in children with cleft palates, the incidence of OME starts to rise around 6 months of age and peaks between 9 months and 1 year. Sanbe states that the peak incidence of serous otitis media in children with cleft palate is between 0-4 years of age, decreasing between 5 to 6 years of age.

It is important to closely monitor and regularly consult with an ENT specialist for any child with a cleft palate, as the early detection and treatment of otitis media with effusion are crucial in preventing long-term hearing issues and complications.

In particular, it is recommended to perform tympanometry regularly, as it is useful for diagnosing the presence of middle ear effusion and whether the middle ear cavity is under negative pressure.

Can I still get otitis media after palatoplasty (cleft palate repair surgery)?

It is widely known that the incidence of otitis media decreases with age for both cleft palate and non-cleft palate children. However, if there is failure in the reconstruction or if the function is poor, the function of the eustachian tube remains inadequate, leading to a higher incidence of otitis media even after surgery. It is speculated that eustachian tube dysfunction will improve as the tube matures with growth. However, if the velar elevator function is impaired, the development of language acquisition can be significantly delayed during crucial developmental periods.

Additionally, if palatoplasty successfully restores the function of the velar elevator, and if nasal-pharyngeal closure is good, the incidence of otitis media with effusion is reduced. That is, successful reconstruction of the velar elevator function improves eustachian tube function, reducing the incidence of otitis media.

Does hearing become difficult?

When a patient develops otitis media, the amount of effusion in the middle ear cavity (middle ear effusion) varies, but it can range from mild conductive hearing loss (around 30-40 dB) to moderate conductive hearing loss of 50-70dB. In many cases, the conductive hearing loss is mild, and around 10% of cases have moderate conductive hearing loss.

Mild conductive hearing loss makes it difficult to hear whispers, but normal conversations can be heard, so it is thought that there is little risk of delayed language development. However, in cases of moderate conductive hearing loss, normal conversation may not be heard clearly.

The lower relative amount of verbal information due to hearing loss can create significant handicaps in language acquisition and emotional development, which requires attention.

What is the difference between otitis media with effusion and acute otitis media?

Otitis media with effusion occurs due to ventilation dysfunction and drainage issues caused by eustachian tube dysfunction. In children, otitis media with effusion is often asymptomatic, which is characteristic of this condition. In contrast, acute otitis media is associated with upper respiratory tract infections and related diseases. The middle ear cavity, connected to the eustachian tube and the upper respiratory tract, can get infected via the eustachian tube, leading to acute otitis media. Most cases of acute otitis media are bacterial infections, and symptoms include strong ear pain (**Fig. 2**).

Both otitis media with effusion and acute otitis media are closely related to the eustachian tube and do not occur via the external auditory canal (**Fig. 1, 2**).

CHAPTER 8. EAR PROBLEMS

Severity classification of acute otitis media in children

First examination score			
Under 2 years old			③

1. Otorrhea	0	1	2
2. Fever (37.0 C)	0	1	2
3. Crying and bad mood	0	①	2

1. Redness of the eardrum	0	②	4
2. Tympanic membrane prominence	0	4	⑧
3. Otorrhea	0	4	8
4. Light cone	0	④	

Total 18 points

Rating: Mild: 0-9 points, Moderate: 10-15 points;
Severe: 16 points or more

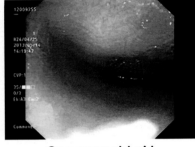

One year old girl weight 7.6 kg

Ozex granules 90mg 2x (7) MA

① Drug name	BLNAR	③ Drug name	PSSP
AMPC	R＞2	AMPC	S＜=0.25
CMX	S＜=0.5	CMX	S＜=0.5
CDTR	S＜=0.5	CDTR	S＜=0.5
CFPM	R2	CFPM	S＜=0.5
CAM	S＜=4	CAM	R＞0.5
AZM	S＜=1	AZM	R＞2
FOM	R128	FOM	R＜=64
TFLX	S＜=0.5	TFLX	S＜=0.5
MUP	R	MUP	R
FRPM	R＞1	FRPM	S＜=0.5

Fig. 2 The eardrum is bulging due to suppuration, a condition that causes intense otalgia

Treatment and precautions in daily life

As a conservative treatment approach, since otitis media with effusion is caused by ventilation dysfunction and drainage problems of the eustachian tube, it is essential to visit an otolaryngologist for nasal treatment and nebulizer therapy.

To improve ventilation, nasal suctioning should be performed adequately to remove nasal discharge, and then the infection-fighting immunity will increase. As the eustachian tube develops with growth, eustachian tube function improves.

In terms of pharmacological treatment: Macrolide antibiotics like clarithromycin have antimicrobial effects and also reduce secretion from inflamed mucosa. Long-term administration of clarithromycin and carbocysteine to improve mucosal function is effective.

If middle ear effusion persists, tympanotomy (myringotomy) is recommended.

The term "incision" may sound alarming, evoking thoughts such as "Is it painful?" or "Is it scary?"

However, when iontophoresis is used in combination with tympanic membrane anesthesia, myringotomy can be performed with minimal to no pain.

Furthermore, if otitis media with effusion recurs frequently or if myringotomy is performed but middle ear effusion reappears within a few days, this can be addressed by placing a ventilation tube in the tympanic membrane (tympanostomy tube) (**Fig. 3**).

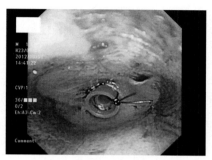

Fig. 3　Inserted ventilation tube

Additionally, if watery or purulent nasal discharge occurs, it is important to visit an otolaryngologist early, where nasal procedures will adequately suction and remove the discharge. Nasal treatment is effective in reducing the bacterial load in nasal discharge, making it very useful in preventing otitis media. In daily life, the most important precaution is not to facilitate negative pressure in the middle ear cavity. Therefore, "sniffing" should be avoided as it can exacerbate this condition.

References
1) Kobayashi K. Cleft palate children. JOHNS, 30 (1): 89-91, 2014.
2) Sasaki Y., Iino Y. Cleft palate children and otitis media. JOHNS, 10 (5): 669-672, 2003.
3) Sanbe T. Cleft palate and otitis media with effusion. Otolaryngology and Head & Neck Surgery, MOOK 11: 74-79, Kanehara Publishing, Tokyo, 1989.

CHAPTER 8. EAR PROBLEMS

Q 117. I WOULD LIKE TO HAVE A HEARING TEST. FROM WHAT AGE IS IT POSSIBLE TO UNDERGO THE TEST?

A There are several types of tests available, so please refer to the following.

In the School Health and Safety Act, it is specified that an audiometer must be used for hearing screening during school entrance exams from around the age of 5 to 6. For children under a certain age, such as those with hearing difficulties, physiological and objective hearing tests, such as Auditory Evoked Potentials (AEP), are recommended. As children grow older, hearing screenings for school entry are conducted using an audiometer. Screening for the presence or absence of hearing is recommended using Otoacoustic Emissions (OAE). However, these screenings primarily focus on a child's response to sound and do not reflect overall hearing ability.

For hearing tests that rely on conditioning, such as the COR test, it can be performed on infants from around 6 months of age. However, COR testing alone is limited, and hearing in both ears cannot be assessed separately. Additionally, tests such as the Play Audiometry Test or Visual Reinforcement Audiometry (VRA) may be appropriate for children at a certain age.

Simple methods like Conditioned Orientation Response (COR) may no longer be sufficient as the child matures. Therefore, at around age 3, objective hearing tests become appropriate for children. Objective tests include Auditory Brainstem Response (ABR) and Otoacoustic Emissions (OAE), which can be used in infants.

However, in certain cases where ABR or OAE tests are desired, it is necessary to confirm in advance whether the facility has the equipment, as these tests may not be available at all medical institutions. University hospitals, pediatric centers, and children's hospitals often possess equipment for more advanced testing, such as Auditory Steady-State Response (ASSR), which can measure hearing thresholds across frequencies from brainwave responses.

References

1) Kobayashi H. Cleft palate children. JOHNS, 30 (1): 89-91, 2014.

2) Mori M. Illustrated Otolaryngology. Bunkodo, Tokyo, 2014, 6-56.

[Q] 118. DOES HAVING A CLEFT PALATE AFFECT THE SENSE OF SMELL?

[A] **There is no direct abnormality in the sense of smell, but it is important to keep the nasal vestibule and nasal cavity clean to prevent acute rhinitis and acute sinusitis.**

The nose and sinuses have several important functions, including warming, humidifying, dust removal, and increasing the intake of oxygen, all of which are essential for breathing. Additionally, the nose is responsible for the sense of smell. Most of the mucous membranes inside the nose are involved in respiration, but the olfactory epithelium, which is responsible for smell, is found only in the olfactory cleft, located in the uppermost part of the nasal cavity.

Therefore, having a cleft palate does not directly lead to abnormalities in the sense of smell. However, if a bacterial infection occurs in the nasal cavity, it can cause inflammation that may extend to the olfactory cleft. This inflammation could potentially damage the olfactory epithelium, resulting in olfactory dysfunction.

To prevent this, it is important to maintain cleanliness in the nasal vestibule and nasal cavity in order to prevent conditions like acute rhinitis and acute sinusitis.

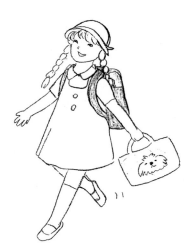

CHAPTER 8. EAR PROBLEMS

Q 119. IS IT TRUE THAT CHILDREN WITH CLEFT LIP AND PALATE HAVE A FOUL-SMELLING NOSE?

A **This is not typically the case. However, in rare instances, a foul odor may develop.**

It is not only children with cleft lip and palate who may have a foul-smelling nose. However, sometimes, food particles may enter the nasal cavity, particularly if the nasal shape, external nose, and nostrils are not properly maintained. In such cases, using a closure device can help prevent unpleasant odors.

In children, if there is an upper respiratory tract infection and bacteria like *Haemophilus influenzae* proliferate in the nasal discharge, an unpleasant nasal odor may occur. To prevent this, cotton balls placed in the nostrils can help control the bacterial growth and avoid odor.

Also, if bacteria like *Streptococcus pneumoniae* or *Haemophilus influenzae* colonize the nasal area, it can cause unpleasant odors, as *Haemophilus influenzae* produces an enzyme that facilitates the generation of the odorant compound indole.

Therefore, caution is necessary when using nasal items, such as cotton or silicone nasal retainer, as they can lead to bacterial growth if they trap nasal discharge. Furthermore, if a child has a cleft palate fistula, the risk of infection increases, which may contribute to odor. In rare cases, *MRSA* (methicillin-resistant *Staphylococcus aureus*) may lead to toxic shock syndrome, caused by toxins produced by the bacteria. For this reason, it is not recommended to use certain nasal devices unless advised by an ENT specialist.

162

CHAPTER *9.* DENTAL PROBLEMS

CHAPTER 9. DENTAL PROBLEMS

Q 120. ARE CHILDREN WITH CLEFT LIP AND PALATE MORE PRONE TO CAVITIES?

A **Yes, they are indeed more susceptible. However, there are reports indicating that children with cleft lip and palate who started oral care early had fewer cavities compared to other children. Therefore, it is crucial to provide oral health guidance and appropriate treatment through regular checkups as they grow.**

Children with cleft lip and palate may face challenges with oral hygiene and dental health. Post-surgical outcomes often lead to improved function, enabling better dietary intake. However, due to the presence of scar tissue, natural cleansing mechanisms can be compromised, especially in areas near the cleft. Teeth adjacent to the cleft tend to tilt, and enamel hypoplasia—the underdevelopment of the enamel layer—is frequently observed. These factors make them more prone to dental caries. Moreover, as children with cleft lip and palate grow and their diet expands to include more solid and sweet foods around 1 year and 6 months, maintaining proper oral hygiene becomes increasingly difficult. Inconsistent feeding schedules, prolonged breastfeeding, and irregular oral cleaning practices can further increase the risk of plaque accumulation and cavities. For this reason, it is essential to establish consistent oral hygiene habits, including brushing, and to ensure regular dental checkups and preventive care.

Healthy oral hygiene practices should be integrated into daily routines, emphasizing regulated meal times and reducing the intake of sugary foods and drinks. By the time the second primary molars erupt (around 3 years old), children experience functional dental development. Early-onset caries, if left unchecked, can progress rapidly, interfering with subsequent speech therapy, orthodontic treatments, and maxillary bone growth. Reports indicate that children who begin oral care early are less likely to develop cavities than their peers. Educating caregivers about proper oral care, coupled with consistent guidance through checkups, plays a vital role in fostering long-term oral health in children with cleft lip and palate, especially after the age of three.

References

1) Toki Y. et al. Management status of children with cleft lip and palate in primary dentition at our pediatric dentistry department. Jpn J Ped Dent, 35 (3): 489-498, 1977.

2) Takahashi S. Fundamentals and Clinical Practice of Cleft Lip and Palate. 1st ed. Nihon Shika Hyoronsha, Tokyo, 1996, 575-578.

Q 121. ARE THERE ANY SPECIAL CONSIDERATIONS WHEN BRUSHING THE TEETH OF CHILDREN WITH CLEFT LIP AND PALATE?
COULD YOU ALSO EXPLAIN THE EFFECTIVENESS OF FLUORIDE IN PREVENTING CAVITIES?

A The details are provided below.

About tooth brushing

It is important to understand the oral environment after surgery for children with cleft lip and palate, as well as how to choose and use a toothbrush. If you brush without considering these factors, children who experience pain while brushing may develop a dislike for brushing or may avoid it altogether.

Regarding when to start brushing your child's teeth, baby teeth typically begin to emerge around 6-8 months of age. At this point, you can begin using a toothbrush as the teeth start to erupt. During this time, it is essential to help your child get used to the change in posture and the sensations around their mouth through play and physical contact. Therefore, initially, you should smile gently and only wipe the baby teeth with gauze, gradually introducing the toothbrush. You should start using a toothbrush only when all four front teeth have fully grown.

For toothbrushes for infants and toddlers, we recommend those with a head approximately the length of two upper primary front teeth, with short, dense, elastic bristles and a low center of gravity (**Fig. 1**). Brushes with bristles that are too long or a head that is too large are unsuitable for infants, as they can damage the gums and make it difficult to clean the cheek and tongue sides of the teeth.

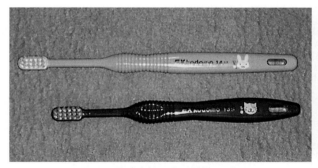
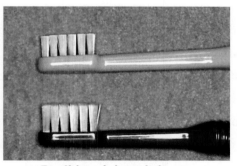

Top: Finishing toothbrush
Bottom: Toddler toothbrush

Toothbrush head shape

Fig. 1 Toothbrushes used in early childhood

For children with a cleft, it is common to bite the brush and spread the bristles. Therefore, we recommend having a separate toothbrush for finishing brushing. Additionally, if cleaning a baby

165

tooth adjacent to an alveolar cleft is difficult with a regular toothbrush, you can use a single-tufted toothbrush (**Fig. 2**), which is ideal for more detailed cleaning.

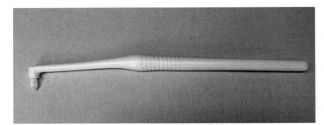

Fig. 2   A single-tufted toothbrush

It is more effective to replace the toothbrush when the bristles have lost their elasticity, rather than when they have become spread apart.

Brushing teeth for children with cleft lip and palate

When brushing a child's teeth, place the toothbrush at a right angle to their teeth and move it back and forth in a quick, vibrating motion about 10 times. The key is to keep the bristles of the toothbrush in one place and gently press them against the tooth surface, allowing the bristles to reach the spaces between the teeth and the area where the teeth meet the gums (**Fig. 3**).

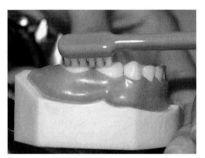

Fig. 3   Place the brush at right angles to teeth

It is important for children to begin brushing their teeth on their own with adult supervision. However, when they are just starting to walk, if they play with a toothbrush in their mouth, they may fall and injure their mouth, so be careful when handing a toothbrush to a child.

Once all baby teeth have grown and the teeth are in close contact with each other, children over the age of 3 can start using floss to clean between the teeth and in areas that cannot be reached with a toothbrush. When inserting floss between the teeth, be careful not to damage the gums, and be sure to remove plaque from both adjacent surfaces.

When children enter elementary school, the first molars (6-year molars) begin to erupt. As new permanent teeth continue to emerge, they have not yet reached the biting surface, making it very difficult to brush them properly. For this reason, it is difficult for children to brush their teeth completely by themselves. Therefore, it is important to encourage them and monitor their brushing, they need adult support.

About fluoride

Fluoride is effective in preventing tooth decay because it enhances the acid resistance of teeth, strengthens enamel, inhibits the progression of tooth decay, promotes remineralization, and reduces the activity of bacteria that cause decay. In Japan, systemic application through the fluoridation of tap water is not practiced, so only local application is used. Fluoride is applied at dental clinics, and toothpaste and mouthwash are used at home, but each method has a different purpose and mechanism of action for prevention. Fluoride application at dental clinics uses high-concentration fluoride (9000 ppm) to improve the acid resistance of enamel, while low-concentration fluoride preparations (225-1000 ppm), such as toothpaste and mouthwashes, are used at home.

By maintaining low concentrations of fluoride in the oral environment for extended periods, we aim to inhibit the progression of tooth decay and promote remineralization.

Fluoride application

The local application of fluoride in infants and toddlers begins when the maxillary deciduous anterior teeth erupt, around age 1, strengthening immature enamel. The frequency of application is typically twice a year when the risk of cavities is low, and can be increased depending on the cavity risk. When children reach school age, the permanent teeth (including anterior teeth, deciduous teeth, and molars) erupt continuously. Therefore, regular fluoride application at a dental clinic is effective in strengthening tooth structure and has been reported to reduce tooth decay by 20-40%.

About fluoride toothpaste

Currently, fluoride toothpaste accounts for 88% of the toothpaste market share in Japan (2005). The rate at which fluoride toothpaste can prevent tooth decay is said to be 20-40%, but its effectiveness varies greatly depending on the method of rinsing after brushing. To enhance the effectiveness of the toothpaste, it is recommended to rinse your mouth with a small amount of water after brushing your teeth.

About fluoride mouth rinse

This is typically introduced around the age of 4, when children can control rinsing and spitting out after 30 seconds. Children with clefts may have difficulty gargling with their lips closed, so it is important to work on improving lip movement through exercises, such as playing with their lips by blowing a flute or inflating balloons. The preventive effect is even greater if fluoride mouthwash is used in addition to toothpaste. Fluoride mouthwash is also used in settings beyond the home, such as nursery schools, kindergartens, and elementary schools, where it has been reported to have a cavity prevention rate of 30-50%. However, over-the-counter fluoride mouthwashes for home use are not available, so a prescription from a dentist is required.

Reference

1) Takaesu Y. et.al. Science of Clinical Application of Fluoride for Dentists and Dental Hygienists in the 21st Century. 1st ed. Nagasue Shoten, Kyoto, 2002, 30, 36, 40.

CHAPTER 9. DENTAL PROBLEMS

[Q] 122. IS SEVERE TEETH GRINDING AFFECTING MY TEETH? IS THERE A WAY TO STOP IT?

[A] **Severe teeth grinding can cause tooth wear, fractures, sensitivity, and gum recession. However, bruxism is considered a physiological behavior that occurs unconsciously, and it is believed to help control various functional and psychological stresses.**

Teeth grinding, also known as bruxism, can affect your child's teeth by causing wear, fractures, tooth sensitivity, and even gum recession. This behavior is often unconscious, especially during sleep, and is usually a way of coping with physical or psychological stress. While teeth grinding is common in children of all ages, including young children, school-aged children, and adolescents, it is often not noticed by parents because it happens while the child is asleep.

Although the exact causes of teeth grinding are not completely understood, it is believed to be related to factors like stress, misaligned bites, underdeveloped feeding functions, or poor sleep habits. For many children, teeth grinding is simply a physiological response to stress, so it doesn't always cause noticeable dental issues. However, when grinding leads to dental problems, treatments are available. These treatments may include adjusting the bite to relieve pressure on specific teeth, using a splint (a thin plastic plate worn at night) to protect the teeth, or even counseling to address stress.

In recent years, an increase in children's bruxism has been noted, with various factors such as psychological stress, imbalances in the bite, developmental issues in chewing function, and sleep habits being considered as potential causes. However, the exact causes and mechanisms of bruxism remain unclear. A survey conducted among preschool parents found that less than half of the parents recognized their children had bruxism, and dental issues arising from grinding were rare. This suggests that teeth grinding is often an unconscious, physiological behavior that helps control various functional and psychological stresses.

Teeth grinding is due to excessive pressure on the teeth and surrounding tissues, which can lead to tooth wear, fractures, sensitivity, and gum recession. Additionally, nighttime grinding can cause muscle fatigue upon waking, and some children may experience difficulty opening their mouths due to restricted jaw movement.

Since there is no fundamental cure for bruxism, treatment focuses on symptom management when dental issues arise. Common approaches include adjusting the bite, using splint therapy, and counseling. To begin, an oral examination is performed to check if the teeth are interfering during chewing, and if necessary, bite adjustments are made.

Splint therapy involves placing a removable, thin plastic plate on the upper teeth, worn during sleep. This helps reduce abnormal muscle tension and the forces acting on the teeth and surrounding tissues, preventing tooth wear. Reports suggest that after several months of nighttime splint use, bruxism can be reduced. With proper management, splints are considered safe for preventing jaw

168

growth issues in children.

Additionally, evaluating and addressing psychological stress is important in managing bruxism effectively. Methods to stop bruxism include reviewing lifestyle habits and seeking counseling therapy, both of which can be effective in managing stress and preventing further damage to the teeth.

It is also important, as past reports have shown that poor sleep habits due to a shift to a nocturnal lifestyle can increase psychological stress, which may contribute to the onset of bruxism. Therefore, reviewing lifestyle habits and counseling therapy are considered effective methods for managing bruxism. It has been suggested that anxiety may increase psychological stress and contribute to the occurrence of teeth grinding. Anxiety therapy is also considered an effective method for managing bruxism.

References

1) Komatsu T. Bruxism in the deciduous dentition. Japanese Journal of Clinical Dentistry for Children, 15(8): 27-35, 2010.

2) Hachmann A. et al. Efficacy of the nocturnal bite plate in the control of bruxism for 3 to 5year children. J Clin Pediatr Dent, 24: 9-15, 1999.

3) Suwa S. et al. Exploring children's teeth grinding: The effects of sleep and lifestyle habits. Japanese Journal of Clinical Dentistry for Children, 15(8): 36-44, 2010.

4) Laberge L. et al. Development of parasomnias from childhood to early adolescence. Pediatrics, 106: 67-74, 2000.

[Q] 123. DOES GETTING CAVITIES AFFECT PRONUNCIATION?

[A] To speak correctly, not only the tongue and lips but also the teeth are important.

In cases of cleft lip and palate, abnormalities in the shape of the teeth and jaw, as well as misalignment of the teeth, can make it difficult to brush teeth properly, increasing the likelihood of cavities. Additionally, orthodontic treatment is often necessary, and the presence of braces can make brushing even more challenging, further contributing to the development of cavities.

Generally, cavities themselves do not directly affect speech, but secondary issues caused by cavities—such as gaps between the teeth or misalignment—can lead to speech difficulties. For example, gaps in the front teeth or missing teeth can cause air to leak, making it difficult to pronounce sounds like "sa, shi, su, se, so" or "za, ji, zu, ze, zo." Similarly, holes in the back teeth can cause the tongue to get caught, disrupting its movement and negatively affecting speech.

To prevent these issues, it is important not only to treat cavities but also to receive proper oral hygiene guidance from a dentist or dental hygienist tailored to the specific condition, focusing on cavity prevention.

169

CHAPTER 9. DENTAL PROBLEMS

[Q] 124. IS IT POSSIBLE TO APPLY FLUORIDE TREATMENT IN THE CASE OF CLEFT LIP AND PALATE?

[A] **There is no reason to avoid fluoride treatment just because a person has a cleft lip and palate.**

Fluoride treatment can be applied in the same way as for other children.

Fluoride application helps to strengthen the quality of the teeth and can lower the risk of cavities. It is generally safe to receive fluoride treatments, even in the case of cleft lip and palate.

In the case of primary teeth, fluoride treatment can begin from around the time the first milk molars emerge, typically around 1 year 6 months old, and continues as the primary teeth fully emerge, which is usually by around 2 years and 6 months of age. This treatment can prevent cavities in primary teeth and improve the quality of the enamel, making the teeth more resistant to decay caused by acids produced by cavity-causing bacteria. The earlier fluoride is applied, the greater the effect on cavity prevention, particularly for newly erupted teeth. If a child does not have cavities by the time all baby teeth have fully grown at age 2 years and 6 months, the risk of developing cavities later on will be lower.

Regular dental visits and fluoride treatment can also lower the risk of cavities in the permanent teeth later on. As the primary teeth come in and grow fully, fluoride application becomes more effective in preventing decay, and the risk of cavities is significantly reduced.

Q 125. WILL A TOOTH GROW IN THE AREA WHERE THERE WAS A CLEFT?

A If there is a tooth bud, a tooth will grow.

Cleft lip and cleft palate are common, with clefts in the lip (cleft lip), the gum (alveolar cleft), and the palate (cleft palate). In cases where there is a congenital absence of the tooth bud, meaning the tooth never forms, a bridge can be used to support a prosthetic.

The cleft in the gum (alveolar cleft) is particularly significant for tooth eruption. In these cases, bone grafting is typically performed to aid tooth eruption. If the tooth does grow, it may emerge at an abnormal angle or in a horizontal position, known as abnormal eruption.

Bone grafting surgery (alveolar bone grafting) is usually performed around the age of 7 to 11 years to fill the area of the gum cleft with bone. After this procedure, orthodontic treatment can help guide the tooth to its correct position.

In cases where there is a space due to missing teeth, orthodontic treatment can close the gap, or prosthetic treatment can fill the space, resulting in a proper bite. In the past, removable dentures or bridges were used, but now, more often, implants are placed to provide a more stable and functional solution. These treatments not only help restore function but also achieve aesthetically pleasing results.

Prosthetic solutions have evolved, and now, implanting artificial roots in the bone has become a common practice for providing more stable and effective prosthetics for children with clefts.

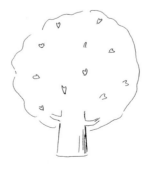

Q 126. PLEASE TEACH ME HOW TO BRUSH TEETH IN THE AREA OF THE ALVEOLAR CLEFT

A **The basic method is to place the bristles of the toothbrush at the boundary between the teeth and the gums and brush gently.**

Teeth near the alveolar cleft are at a higher risk of cavities and periodontal disease due to the quality of the teeth and difficulty cleaning them. Both milk teeth and permanent teeth are crucial for dental treatment, such as orthodontics and alveolar cleft bone grafting, so brushing is very important. Before brushing, check the number of teeth, their orientation, whether any teeth are loose, and if there are any orthodontic devices in place.

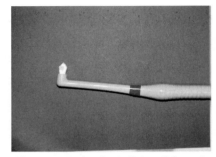

Fig. 1 A single tuft toothbrush

The basic method of brushing is to place the toothbrush bristles at the boundary between the teeth and gums and brush gently. However, it can be difficult to reach these areas, so in those cases, a "single tuft toothbrush" (**Fig. 1**) is recommended as it is easy to maneuver and targets specific spots effectively.

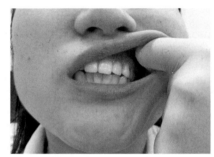

Fig. 2 Creating space

Because of the low amount of supporting bone in cases of bilateral clefts, when teeth are loose, be careful about the pressure applied. Use your hand that isn't holding the toothbrush to support the loose teeth, making sure they don't move too much.

In cases where lip cleft surgery has been performed, the lip may be hardened from scarring, and the oral vestibule (the space between the lips and teeth) may become shallow. When brushing or checking the teeth, it may be necessary to lift the lip, but this could cause pain. In such cases, insert a finger toward the back teeth and lift the lip gently to create space, which will reduce pain (**Fig. 2**).

If food gets stuck in the alveolar cleft (gums), rinse with water, and use a soft toothbrush (preferably an adult-sized one with longer bristles) or a cotton swab to gently remove the food. If it is difficult to remove, avoid forcing it and visit a dental clinic for assistance.

In addition to daily self-care, from a young age, establish a relationship with a regular dentist and prevent cavities and periodontal disease through regular professional care by the dentist and dental hygienist.

[Q] 127. IS IT EASIER TO DEVELOP PERIODONTAL DISEASE IF YOU HAVE A CLEFT LIP AND PALATE?

[A] **Having a cleft lip and palate does not directly make you more susceptible to periodontal disease. However, early use of feeding appliances or orthodontic devices can create an environment where gingivitis is more likely. Therefore, it is important to prevent gingivitis before the completion of orthodontic treatment.**

Having a cleft lip and palate does not directly make you more susceptible to periodontal disease. Periodontal disease occurs when pathogenic bacteria infect the periodontal tissues, and if the immune function is weakened, the surrounding tissues, particularly the alveolar bone, are destroyed. If gingivitis becomes chronic and severe, it can progress into periodontal disease. As a result, the support for the teeth is lost, and in severe cases, tooth mobility and tooth loss can occur. Although periodontal disease can develop in younger individuals, it usually increases significantly after the age of 40.

Children with cleft lip and palate often wear feeding appliances or orthodontic devices from an early age and may have dental anomalies such as malocclusion, dental abnormalities, tooth number anomalies, and tooth position abnormalities, which create an environment that is more prone to gingivitis.

Therefore, it is crucial to regularly attend dental check-ups and practice good oral hygiene, as self-care alone may not be sufficient. Preventing gingivitis before completing orthodontic treatment is essential.

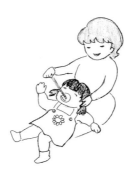

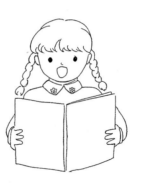

CHAPTER *10.* PSYCHOLOGICAL PROBLEMS

CHAPTER 10. PSYCHOLOGICAL PROBLEMS

Q 128. WHAT IS THE CONSULTATION AND TELEPHONE SUPPORT SYSTEM?

A Contact the Japanese Cleft Palate Foundation, an UN-recognized roster organization.

UN-Recognized Organization (Roster) Japanese Cleft Palate Foundation provides telephone consultation services for professionals and guardians to address their concerns and questions related to cleft lip and palate.

Reception Hours: Monday to Friday, from 10:00-16:00.

After registering, a specialized volunteer doctor will call you back via collected registered call.

You can also send inquiries via letter or email, but telephone consultation is preferred.

Contact Information:

Phone: 052-757-4312

Email: jcpf@jcpf.or.jp

Website: http://www.jcpf.or.jp/

Q 129. WHEN SHOULD I CONSULT A CLINICAL PSYCHOLOGIST?

A If you have any mental health concerns, such as anxiety or worries, feel free to visit and consult them with ease.

When facing problems that you cannot resolve on your own, how reassuring it would be to have someone nearby to consult. "Pray to god when you are in trouble"—in this case, the "god" varies depending on the issue.

If it's a physical health concern, the "god" would likely be a doctor. If it's a matter of human relationships, it might be a lawyer. And if it's about anxiety, worries, or other mental health issues, then a clinical psychologist would be your "god."

Experts with specialized knowledge and skills can help resolve difficult problems. However, in Japan, aside from doctors and lawyers, there is often hesitation to consult a clinical psychologist. Some believe that seeking such help is only for "weak" or "special" individuals, which can lead to reluctance in reaching out.

As a result, many people bear the burden of their emotional struggles alone, prolonging their suffering and, in some cases, leading to mental illness. Consulting a specialist when faced with a

176

problem can provide a fresh perspective, a new way of thinking, or a different approach, which often brings relief.

Those who seek help from professionals during challenging times are not weak; on the contrary, they demonstrate strength. As the saying goes, "It is easier done than said." With a bit of courage and an open mind, you can visit a clinical psychologist for support.

For more details, please refer to the website of the Japanese Clinical Psychologists Association listed below.

Reference

1) How to connect with a clinical psychologist. http://www.jsccp.jp/near/

Q 130. HOW CAN BULLYING BE PREVENTED OR ERADICATED?

A Efforts are being made to prevent bullying through the development of strategic language programs and other measures. For cases of severe bullying, do not struggle alone—consider reaching out to a hotline for free counseling and support.

Even though the single word "bullying" is used, it encompasses a variety of cases. Some children may find themselves isolated within their group of friends, while others may be targeted by a specific child. In some instances, not only the individual but even their siblings may become targets of bullying. For the individual and their parents, bullying can bring immense humiliation and sadness. However, the lessons learned from such experiences can serve as a foundation for personal growth and resilience.

Addressing bullying is critical, and the solutions will depend on the situation and the individual's personality. Helping the person communicate their feelings is essential. If speaking up is difficult, writing down their experiences to convey the pain of being bullied is a constructive approach. Teachers can also play a significant role by providing detailed explanations about cleft lip and palate, including the days when the student may need to miss school for medical appointments. This can foster understanding and empathy among classmates. Teaching children that making comments about others' appearances is unacceptable is another way to dismantle societal prejudices and encourage the development of empathy.

At our facility, the goal of treatment goes beyond surgery and speech therapy to help children integrate better with their peers. Our focus is on nurturing the child into a person who excels in areas where they have put in effort. For example, in speech therapy, we not only teach the child to speak normally but also incorporate methods that promote intellectual development. This helps children acquire knowledge beyond their peers, build self-confidence, and recognize their strengths. With

CHAPTER 10. PSYCHOLOGICAL PROBLEMS

this foundation, even if they face occasional bullying, they can understand and embrace their unique qualities, earning respect from others.

We also use strategic language programs to prevent bullying and foster positive social interactions. Orthodontic and implant treatments further contribute by improving dental alignment, allowing children to have better teeth and a more confident smile compared to their peers or even family members.

For cases of severe bullying, the Japanese Cleft Palate Foundation provides a support system, offering professional advice from lawyers and clinical psychologists. A hotline is also available for free consultations (excluding phone charges). Additionally, the Japanese Cleft Palate Foundation publishes resources such as booklets for teachers during enrollment and when children enter elementary school, along with a booklet of mothers' experiences to guide families through these challenges.

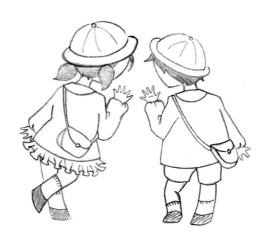

CHAPTER *11.* OTHERS

CHAPTER 11. OTHERS

Q 131. HOW DO THE GENERAL PUBLIC RECOGNIZE SPEECH DISORDERS RELATED TO CLEFT LIP AND CLEFT PALATE?

A It is necessary to take measures early as possible.

Previous research has reported that the general public tends to evaluate speech disorders related to cleft palate negatively. However, there are still many unknowns regarding how the general public perceives cleft palate speech.

In recent studies, Hayakawa et al. analyzed the auditory perception of cleft palate speech among the general public, exploring the impressions it creates. According to their findings, most people were able to correctly distinguish between cleft palate speech and normal speech. Moreover, while they held negative impressions of cleft palate speech, they also expressed some positive perceptions.

Achieving speech that closely resembles normal sound requires long-term speech training. The negative impressions associated with cleft palate speech can affect a child's psychosocial development. Therefore, it is essential to take early measures to improve the perceptions of others. In this regard, Makino et al. reported that modifying the speech rate of cleft palate speech could be useful. Future research is expected to lead to the development of new training methods alongside traditional speech training to acquire correct pronunciation.

References
1) Hayakawa T. et al. Perception of cleft palate speech by Japanese listeners. Aichi-Gakuin Dent Sci, 23: 15-29, 2010.
2) Makino H. et al. The perception of cleft palate speech by variations in speed first report: Articulation distortion from nasal emission. Aichi-Gakuin Dent Sci, 25: 9-16, 2012.

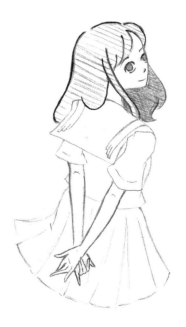

Q 132. IS IT POSSIBLE TO EXPERIENCE DISCRIMINATION DURING EMPLOYMENT OR MARRIAGE?

A It is possible, but it is important to make efforts to overcome such challenges.

Unfortunately, it is not possible to completely deny the possibility of discrimination. However, it is a fact that everyone faces various challenges. The first step is to understand and accept your own condition, and then make efforts to help those around you understand naturally as well.

If you are concerned about employment or marriage, it is a good idea to seek advice. You can take advantage of the free phone consultation service provided by the Japanese Cleft Palate Foundation. Many experienced experts are available to offer advice, and they can also connect you with a consulting lawyer if needed. Additionally, if desired, they can introduce you to individuals who have gone through similar experiences, including cleft lip and palate patients and their families.

No one is perfect. Instead of giving up because of a medical condition, it is important to make the effort to overcome it.

Q 133. WHEN A POTENTIAL PARTNER FOR MARRIAGE APPEARS, SHOULD YOU TELL THEM ABOUT YOUR CLEFT LIP AND PALATE?

A Yes, you should tell them, but there are also ways to specifically consult on how to explain it.

Of course, you should explain cleft lip and palate in an easy-to-understand way. Before that, it is necessary to understand the condition properly yourself. In addition to various books, there are methods available for consulting specifically on how to explain it, such as genetic counseling or phone consultations with the Japanese Cleft Palate Foundation.

If you wish to consult, please contact the Japanese Cleft Palate Foundation (TEL: 052-757-4312) between Monday and Friday from 10:00 AM to 4:00 PM. A specialist volunteer will call you back later. Please note that genetic counseling is a paid service.

CHAPTER 11. OTHERS

Q 134. AS A PATIENT WITH CLEFT LIP AND PALATE, YOU MAY WANT TO HAVE A PARTNER OR GET MARRIED, BUT YOU MIGHT WORRY THAT YOUR APPEARANCE OR GENETIC CONCERNS WILL EVENTUALLY DISAPPOINT YOUR PARTNER, MAKING YOU FEEL THAT YOU CANNOT BE "THE BEST PARTNER" FOR THEM. WHAT SHOULD YOU DO?

A **By being able to consider things from your partner's perspective, you have the potential to become the best partner for them.**

After many years of treating patients with cleft lip and palate, I have found that many are "kind" and "gentle," and many are also "filial." No one is perfect in every aspect. I believe that understanding yourself and striving to be a good partner for someone else are essential. It is also important to study and work diligently so that you can be recognized and valued by those around you.

Your ability to consider things from the perspective of others gives you the potential to be the best partner for them. Instead of focusing solely on finding a romantic partner, it is crucial to cultivate empathy for everyone, regardless of age or gender. Through this, meaningful connections will arise.

Q 135. IF THE PERSON YOU DECIDED TO MARRY, OR THEIR FAMILY, HAS CLEFT LIP AND PALATE, AND YOU ARE CONSIDERING BREAKING OFF THE MARRIAGE DUE TO PARENTAL OPPOSITION, WHAT SHOULD YOU DO?

A **Marriage is about overcoming various challenges together and living life as partners.**

The occurrence of cleft lip and palate in the children of those affected is very rare. Please approach this with scientific knowledge and make a calm, rational decision. Everyone has a different susceptibility to conditions such as cancer or neurological diseases.

If you consider giving up on a marriage due to minor issues, you may find yourself facing multi-

182

ple divorces throughout your life. Marriage is about overcoming various challenges and living life together.

The Japanese Cleft Palate Foundation offers free consultations. Additionally, if you wish to learn more, genetic counseling with an expert (for a fee) is available to discuss hereditary matters.

[Q] 136. I SAW A TV BROADCAST SHOWING CHILDREN FROM DEVELOPING COUNTRIES WITH CLEFT LIPS, AND MY CHILD STARTED CRYING. IS IT ETHICALLY ACCEPTABLE FOR TV STATIONS TO AIR SUCH FOOTAGE?

[A] If there is an issue, it is important to raise concerns with the TV station and ask for reflection.

There have been reports of children being bullied by their classmates in elementary school in Japan after seeing close-up images of unoperated children's cleft lips on TV. Unfortunately, it is a sad reality that many TV staff prioritize attracting viewers' attention over ethical considerations. If an issue arises, it is important to raise the matter with the TV station and ask for reflection. It is crucial to communicate that the content was uncomfortable.

The Japanese Cleft Palate Foundation addresses such issues by raising concerns with TV stations, publishers, and others when necessary. In these cases, please contact them with objective information, such as recordings.

[Q] 137. IT IS SOMETIMES SEEN THAT OLDER INDIVIDUALS HAVE SCARS ON THEIR UPPER LIPS. IS IT POSSIBLE TO TREAT THIS EVEN NOW?

[A] With the latest medical advancements, it is highly likely that improvement is possible.

Medical advancements have been remarkable, and with improvements in surgical techniques and post-operative care, it is highly likely that even individuals who underwent surgery many years ago can achieve significant improvements.

CHAPTER 11. OTHERS

The possibility of improving the condition is high with current medical technologies.

Q 138. MY BOYFRIEND, WHO HAS A CLEFT LIP AND PALATE, INTERRUPTED HIS TREATMENT WHEN HE WAS YOUNG, AND IS NOW 20 YEARS OLD.
IT IS LIKELY THAT SURGERY COULD IMPROVE HIS CONDITION, BUT HE IS NOT UNDERGOING THE PROCEDURE.
ADDITIONALLY, HE HAS POOR DENTAL ALIGNMENT, CAVITIES, AND HAS RECENTLY STARTED TO NOTICE BAD BREATH. WHAT SHOULD BE DONE?

A **Rather than pushing for surgery right away, it might be a good idea for him to undergo a regular check-up to assess whether there are any current issues that need attention.**

For individuals with cleft lip and palate, many people feel that it is okay to be their true selves as they are.

If you're encouraging him to resume treatment, it's important to do so in a way that doesn't hurt his feelings. Instead of focusing on urging surgery, perhaps it would be better to recommend regular check-ups to assess whether there are any current issues.

If bad breath is a concern, it could be due to conditions related to the cleft lip and palate, but it's also possible that other health issues might be discovered.

Q 139. PLEASE TELL ME ABOUT THE JAPANESE CLEFT PALATE FOUNDATION

A **Please refer to the following.**

The Japanese Cleft Palate Foundation was established in 1 January, 1992 as a non-profit volunteer organization. Through membership, individuals gain access to various services and information re-

184

garding cleft lip and palate, as well as resources such as a cleft lip and palate hotline and medical aid in various countries.

Founded with the aim of supporting the healthy development of children with congenital cleft lip and palate, the association is active through the efforts of medical professionals, patients, healthcare workers, businesses, and the general public. It holds the distinction of being Japan's largest organization dedicated to cleft lip and palate.

The association is a registered non-profit organization (NPO), recognized by the government as a public service entity, and is qualified to offer tax-deductible donations.

The Japanese Cleft Palate Foundation engages in various activities, including publishing newsletters on cleft lip and palate, hosting lectures and film screenings, offering genetic counseling related to cleft lip and palate, and operating a remote speech and language trainings.
For more information, visit our website.
http://www.jcpf.or.jp/

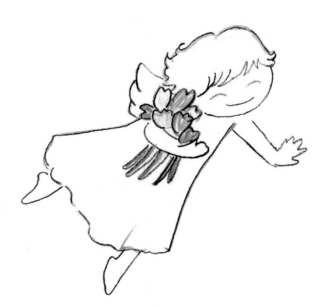

CHAPTER 11. OTHERS

Q 140. PLEASE TELL ME ABOUT THE INTERNATIONAL CLEFT LIP AND PALATE FOUNDATION: ICPF

A Please refer to the following.

The International Cleft Lip and Palate Foundation (ICPF) was established in Kyoto on 23 October 1997, by the late Professor David Precious of Dalhousie University in Canada and Professor Nagato Natsume of Aichi Gakuin University, Japan. It is an international humanitarian organization that focuses on the treatment of cleft lip and palate, which are among the most common congenital abnormalities, occurring in 1 in 500 to 1,000 births in Japan, and affecting more than 14 million people worldwide.

ICPF has a team of surgeons, orthodontists, speech therapists, geneticists, pediatricians, anesthesiologists, and other medical professionals essential for ensuring that patients receive appropriate treatment. The team also includes the patients themselves and their families. As of May 2015, our membership numbered approximately 2,400, representing various regions and countries, making us one of the leading international organizations specializing in cleft lip and palate.

The ICPF aims to ensure that children worldwide receive proper treatment for cleft lip and palate, enabling them to grow up healthy. Unfortunately, in developing and impoverished countries, children with cleft lip and palate often cannot access medical professionals capable of performing the necessary surgeries, leading to discrimination and neglect. This sad reality is largely due to a lack of societal awareness and understanding, as well as prejudice against those with the condition.

ICPF works to improve this situation by promoting education and knowledge about cleft lip and palate, advocating for greater understanding within societies, and focusing on training medical professionals in developing countries so they can provide appropriate treatment. This is considered a key goal, as it allows these countries to provide the same standard of care seen in developed nations.

ICPF also coordinates free surgeries and shares information with medical professionals in these countries to assist them in learning and adopting proper treatment techniques. The foundation hopes that through continued efforts, children with cleft lip and palate, regardless of where they are born, will one day have access to the necessary treatment.

For more information on ICPF and their activities, please refer to the ICPF website: http://www.icpfweb.org/about/index. html or ICPF Facebook page.

Editor
Nagato Natsume

Authors
Yoshiko Aihara

Junko Akashi

Kumiko Fujiwara

Takuya Fujiwara

Hiroo Furukawa

Toko Hayakawa

Kensuke Hayashi

Hideto Imura

Chisako Inoue

Hiyori Makino

Katsuhiro Minami

Ken Miyazawa

Tomoko Mori

Hiroshi Murakami

Nagana Natsume

Nagato Natsume

Hiroyuki Nawa

Teruyuki Niimi

Naoki Saito

Tatsunori Shibazaki

Yoshitaka Toyama

Maya Yoshida

Translated by
Tselmuun Chinzorig

Oyunaa Erdene

Ariuntuul Garidkhuu

Duurenjargal Myagmarsuren